TANTRA 2.0

Modern Interpretations of an Ancient Yoga

CHAITANYA PRABHU HAKKALADADDI

notionpress.com

INDIA · SINGAPORE · MALAYSIA

Copyright © Chaitanya Prabhu Hakkaladaddi 2023
All Rights Reserved.

ISBN 979-8-89133-976-7

This book has been published with all efforts taken to make the material error-free after the consent of the author. However, the author and the publisher do not assume and hereby disclaim any liability to any party for any loss, damage, or disruption caused by errors or omissions, whether such errors or omissions result from negligence, accident, or any other cause.

While every effort has been made to avoid any mistake or omission, this publication is being sold on the condition and understanding that neither the author nor the publishers or printers would be liable in any manner to any person by reason of any mistake or omission in this publication or for any action taken or omitted to be taken or advice rendered or accepted on the basis of this work. For any defect in printing or binding the publishers will be liable only to replace the defective copy by another copy of this work then available.

Contents

About the Author 5
Book Preview 7

Tantra 2.0 9
    Introduction 10
    How to Use This Book 14

Body 16
    Shatkriyas—Caring for the Body 16
    Asanas—Yoga Postures 19
    Bandhas—Body Locks 20

The 5 Fives—Systems of Reality 23
    5 Layers of Self 24
    5 States of Awareness 25
    5 Powers of God 28
    5 Acts of God 30
    5 Veils of Ignorance 32

Mind & Consciousness 35
    36 Tattvas 43
    The Occult Tattvas 52
    Tantra Meditation.. 57
    Buddhist Meditation 61
    Becoming Gods 70
    Raja Yoga (Patanjali's Yoga Sutras): The Eightfold Path........... 72

Epilogue—Tantric Sex & Kundalini.. *87*
Book Preview *92*

About the Author

I started my career in Molecular Biology but moved on to Computer Journalism and ended up in Instructional Design and Learning Consultancy. However, my interest in the Science of Consciousness persisted. Over 25 years of writing (as a Journalist and Learning Consultant) puts me in a unique position to write about Tantra from a scientific perspective.

I started practicing Yoga almost 30 years ago and learned how yogic postures help us communicate with our bodies. Then I practiced Tantra and learned that Yoga is about stretching, contorting the muscles, and exercising the mind.

At that time, I was the Editor of a men's magazine, which gave me ample scope to explore tantric sex besides studying its Philosophy. A few years ago, I practiced Yoga under a Tantrik Guru, which motivated me to write this book.

I present Tantra 2.0 as a simple guide to the practice of Tantra Yoga. I have avoided "divinity" and "spirituality" as much as possible because of their vagueness. I have also avoided symbolism, which is irrelevant in our technological times. For example, what symbolic meaning does the lotus plant convey to you? It means nothing to me!

Similarly, suppose the symbolic artifacts of Yantras and Mandalas are not already pre-existing in your socio-cultural context. In that case, they are of no use in the comprehension and practice of Tantra.

I have avoided references to esoteric interpretations, highlighted the garbage that Google spews out, and pointed out the fatalistic and dehumanizing nature of religions.

However, I must confess that my efforts may not have been enough.

Chaitanya Prabhu Hakkaladaddi

Book Preview

Vigyan Bhairava Tantra: Modern Interpretations of the Conversations between Kali and Shiva

Note to the Reader

Writing this book has been a pleasure, and the journey has been easy. However, it has not been as easy to get people to realize the relevance of Tantra in the modern world.

In this context, I request you—the reader—to assist me by leaving me a review offering any constructive criticism or feedback for improvements.

Your suggestions will be highly appreciated. Please send your feedback to lightandgracebooks@gmail.com

Also by Chaitanya

Kundalini Awakening: 8 Pathways to Enlightenment

Coming soon:

Vigyan Bhairava Tantra: Modern Interpretation of the Conversations between Kali and Shiva

Tantra 2.0

Tantra reveals itself slowly through practice. It is not a belief system, religion, or doctrine. It provides techniques—techniques that one may use for Good or Evil.

When Tantra reveals itself through Yoga, it does so through experiences unique to each individual. Most of these experiences are explainable through a common language, but many are not. Cognitively, these experiences are novel, arising from an altered consciousness, involving unusual sensations and uncommon manifestations.

On rare occasions, they may be similar to those witnessed in the clinically insane or those under the influence of drugs/alcohol. We cannot identify with these experiences, so we categorize them as strange, mystical, or occult.

However, when we practice established tantric processes, we comprehend these perfectly healthy (but altered) states of the mind.

Mantra, Mystery, Magic? Not Really!

More like… Psychology, Process, Practice!

Introduction

Tantra is one of the many spiritual traditions of ancient India, which influenced Hinduism and Buddhism. It comprises many diverse traditions, and each tantric practice has the awakening of consciousness or achieving enlightenment at its core.

Immediately, I must explain the word "spiritual." Ancient human societies worldwide have identified with "spirits," so "The Spirit" is universal. However, the idea itself is diverse in its interpretation. Some cultures have associated it with a God (theistic), while others associated it with nature (animistic). One also finds many variations between these two extremes—some even deny any such thing as "Spirit."

Here, I will refer to "spiritual" as an experience that is not mundane, not vulgar, and not exclusive to humans (higher-order animals also experience it). Mostly, I will not use the word—overused and abused as it is.

Twenty-five years of tantric practice have taught me that comprehending something means arriving at a state of consciousness. I can "know" a chair in a few nanoseconds, but philosophical subjects take several months or years. However, within the sphere of consciousness, there is no consensus on what consciousness is! No definition is accurate enough, no description is complete, and no explanation is satisfactory.

We popularly agree that it emanates from the mind, but closer examination will show that we are merely conscious of the "concept of mind;" there are different consciousnesses that different body parts can generate.

It may even manifest entirely outside of our bodies! Therefore, consciousness creates the mind and not the other way around! Tantra deals with these manifestations of consciousness—it is not at all concerned with defining them! It is a collection of techniques, tools, and ritualistic processes.

By adhering to these processes—with no prejudices of religion or faith—we can bring the positive, existential benefits we desire.

What is Tantra?

The term is conjured from two Sanskrit words, *Tanoti* and *Trayate,* where *Tanoti* means "to expand" and *Trayate* means "to liberate."

It also owes its meaning to the parts of the word "Tantra," wherein "tan" means the body and "tra" means mechanism or tool. This implies that tantriks use the body as a tool for liberation.

In the dualistic sense, the body is expanding to liberate the mind. This interpretation also works, but the ultimate aim of Tantra is to achieve oneness with reality or to become inseparable from the expanse of universal consciousness.

Tantra destroys this mind-body duality and body-environment, bringing about a communion of the creature with the cosmos.

What Tantra is Not!

Tantra does not mean "to weave" and has nothing to do with the weaving loom. This is a literal—and entirely incorrect—translation by non-Sanskrit, Western experts. For more details, refer to *Tantra Illuminated* by Christopher Wallis (https://hareesh.org).

How to Practice Tantra

I did not have the Internet when I started my Tantra practice about 30 years ago. Therefore, I plowed through libraries and esoteric texts to find some meaningful interpretations of Tantra. However, all I saw were vague or downright silly explanations and discourses of tantric philosophy. Some 20 years ago, things became more accessible with the advent of the Internet, and I began establishing my practices and methodologies.

Here, I share what I did. Firstly, I refused to accept any book that could not explain Tantra in simple, twentieth-century English. My scientific and atheistic temperament would not tolerate any esoteric or religious nonsense!

Secondly, I put the techniques into practice. Regardless of how silly or strange they seemed, I tried them out. If some textbook said, "… go vegetarian to taste the tattva of a food item," then I went vegan for a few months. In that exercise, besides feeling highly energized and sexually stimulated, I also began to "taste" simple food.

Thirdly, I am a trained Molecular Biologist, so my approach to Tantra has been scientific. My motto was, "Explore, observe, be skeptical, challenge the status quo, question the obvious, and trust only reproducible results."

In this context, I could not accept anything dogmatic about Tantra. In addition, as an atheist, I could not take anything religious. Thus, the techniques came to me in a secular fashion. About 20 to 30 years ago, the Western version of Tantra was highly narrow-minded in its focus on sex and did not even offer a peek into the Vama Marga or the Left-Hand Path. Although extremely satisfying, tantric sex was not enough. So, my quest continued…

I gradually realized the Physiology and Psychology behind tantric practices and finally interpreted the tantric texts from a modern, scientific point of view. Add to this Western Occultism and the Science of Consciousness, and we have Tantra 2.0—this book you hold in front of you.

How to Use This Book

The previous pages describe Tantra, its meaning, and its definition in about 1000 words. Each of the paragraphs—and perhaps even each sentence in those paragraphs—can act as a seed for tomes and tomes of debate and discussion. It is not my intention to present a vast encyclopedia of academic research.

Tantra 2.0 succinctly presents the Tantras (several tantric philosophies), cutting through archaic and esoteric language. This book portrays practical techniques anyone interested in the subject can apply. However, it would be best if you acted upon and against" the obsession to comprehend Tantra from a purely academic perspective. Recognize the addiction and realize that it is wasteful.

Tantra is at least 2500 years old. The word Tantra was first found in the Rig Veda, which is now about 3500 years old. Patanjali mentions Tantra, which forms the basis of Buddhism (about 2500 years old). As it grew, practices changed, concepts transformed, and new meanings arose. Hence, there is no absolute, authoritative source of Tantra. In this context, why bother beyond a point?

The more meaningful and satisfying aspects of Tantra are in its daily practice. Therefore, do not be caught up in academic nit-picking—get up (literally) and take action. Tantra Yoga offers an entire philosophy (because Yoga loosely translates as Philosophy) by combining teachings from the ancient Indian Schools of Thought (*Nyaya, Vaisheshika, Samkhya, Yoga, Mimamsa,* and *Vedanta*). When these combinations differed, they gave rise to different traditions, and one of these traditional systems is the Non-Dual Shaiva Tantra (NST) philosophy.

Tantra 2.0 draws upon Non-Dual Shaiva Tantra Philosophy in its interpretations and executions of daily practices. This is the only tradition of Tantra that I have personally found meaningful from a scientific perspective: it appealed to my modern sense of existence.

A Modern Interpretation

In Tantra 2.0, I have combined the practice of Tantra with the Science of Consciousness and Modern Psychology to provide a system of living. I have found parallels between Occult Tantra and modern existential experiences that will be automatically obvious. Additionally, I have explored scientific research into the mind to show "how we think" and "how we perceive reality."

I have presented all this in simple English or through examples from everyday life. My approach is that of a modern man adapting ancient techniques for superior living. Let us enjoy the ride!

Body

"Tan" means the body, and "tra" means mechanism or tool. We use the body as a tool to achieve liberation. Therefore, one interpretation of Tantra can be "Of Body," but this succinctness requires elaboration.

Our existence is nothing more than our body. The mind manifests through the brain, and there is no such thing as the Soul or Spirit. When we realize that we are separate from our biological parents (our creators), the existential question of our identity comes into being. 'God as Creator' is meaningless, and our animal instincts do not need it.

After the umbilical cord is severed (literally and metaphorically), our existence depends on our bodily actions to survive and thrive. Linking our existence to a supernatural entity is the primary purpose of religion. Rather plainly, Tantra abstains from this by stating, "I exist."

By reflecting on my existence, "I exist," I do not justify! "I am." The only proof of my existence is my body.

Shatkriyas—Caring for the Body

Any meaningful discussion of Tantra must discard God (in the conventional and mundane sense, we understand God) and toss the

Soul, Spirit, Holy Ghost, etc. Some even consider these ideas as creations of pompous minds. Our mind is God, our body is the Temple, and righteous action is the Spirit! A firm belief in this statement will make us realize our body is a complex biochemical mass capable of the worst kinds of violence and the highest forms of art.

It is a complex aggregation of parts comprising organs, tissues, and cells. Think of a car; we must care for it like any car. Those who love their cars will comprehend this; those who do not need to realize that you can never overestimate your body.

In this context, Shatkriyas (also called Shatkarmas) are six (shat) cleansing routines:

1. **Trataka**: Cleansing of the eyes

2. **Kapalabhati**: Forceful exhalations to cleanse the lungs and respiratory tract

3. **Neti**: Cleansing of the nasal passage

4. **Dhauti**: Cleansing the stomach

5. **Nauli**: Cleansing the stomach and small intestine

6. **Basti**: Cleansing the large intestine (colonic irrigation)

Instructions for these exercises are pretty simple and easy to understand. However, Neti, Basti, and Dhauti may seem extreme to some Yoga practitioners, so here are the alternatives:

- We can also perform Neti with a Neti Pot (Google it and see if you can buy one online). You can also use any pot with a spout.

Once the water flows into one nostril, it will automatically come out of the other. It does not require much effort.

- You can do Dhauti by drinking lots of lukewarm water (with teardrop salinity). Salinity is essential—you should not be able to taste it after adding salt. Add a little salt. After drinking 2 to 3 glasses, you should be able to induce vomiting (put a finger down your throat or perform Nauli).

- You can perform Basti using your finger instead of a hollow pipe. This is not an extreme option.

Note: The frequency of these Shatkriyas is essential—do not overdo it!

- Trataka (Cleansing of the eyes): 5 to 15 minutes, once daily.

- Kapalabhati (Forceful exhalations): 20 to 100 exhalations, once daily.

- Neti (Cleansing of the nasal passage): Thrice a week.

- Dhauti (Cleansing the stomach): Once a month.

- Nauli (Cleansing the stomach and small intestine): Once daily.

- Basti (Cleansing the large intestine): If you adopt less extreme options once a month or once a week.

Shanka Prakshalana: This intensive cleansing exercise involves the entire digestive system. (You can Google it.) Do this only once every six months. Perform all preparatory actions and take all precautions as if following a medical prescription. The most important instruction is to ensure that you never perform it alone!

Always have someone around during and after the exercise to watch over you!

Asanas—Yoga Postures

Sthirham, Sukham, Asanam! (Sanskrit) means that you must perform all asanas in a balanced and relaxed manner. It is crucial "to have" balance, and you can develop it by being conscious of it. It is also essential "to be" in a relaxed state.

Balance (Sthirham)

Balance is not merely achieving proficiency in the posture of an asana; it is ensuring a balance between the body and breath. When you miss breathing, you miss the essence of Yoga.

Relaxation (Sukham)

Breath also connects with relaxation, but how does one achieve peace in a physically contorted—and often painful—posture? The answer is simple: To perform any relaxation, there cannot be any pain; some discomfort is OK—and even recommended—but there shouldn't be any pain.

We need to manage this by doing the asanas slowly—very slowly; and achieving results over weeks and months, not minutes and days. This ensures no sudden or jerky movements that may cause spasms or sprains. However, what is simple to do is also simple not to do, which is why one sees Yoga performed like aerobics!

T'ai Chi is like Yoga; it is "meditation in motion." Performing Yoga slowly and deliberately acquaints one with one's own body. Close your eyes while doing the asanas and perform the movements slowly, and you will feel as if you are "talking" to your muscles and joints.

Many things can distract you from establishing a connection with your body: uncomfortable clothes, noise, other people, etc., but the most distracting is what many experts recommend—counting! Counting while doing an asana is most distracting because it keeps the mind engaged with the reason, not the body.

Perform the asanas relaxed to achieve a "Balance between Body, Mind, and Breath!"

Bandhas—Body Locks

Bandhas are body locks that correspond to some major sphincters. Traditional Yoga refers to three major Bandhas that I will describe here, but I will also mention some minor bandhas. The concept behind Yogic Bandhas is to control the sphincters. Today, the human body has over 60 types of sphincters. We cannot handle all of them, but we can exert a force on many of them.

1. **Jalandhara Bandha**: Try to press your chin to the upper part of your chest, and you will have achieved this lock. Another way of doing it is to swallow your saliva and not release the throat muscle. This helps to lock the sphincter in your throat.

2. **Uddiyana Bandha**: Exhale profoundly and suck in your stomach. Then, contract your abdominal muscles. This exerts pressure on the junction of the food pipe leading into the stomach.

3. **Mula Bandha**: This locks the excretory sphincters (urinary and fecal). Doing this Bandha is like stopping your urine or contracting your anal sphincter. You may already know that these are two separate sphincters, but while performing this Bandha, it would help if you try to identify them distinctly.

4. **Maha Bandha**: Practicing all the locks simultaneously is Maha Bandha (or the Great Bandha). While leading up to this Bandha, check if you are holding your breath while performing the Mula Bandha. Initially, it is OK if you are, but the correct performance of Mula Bandha is ensuring normal breathing even while in Mula Bandha. It will be evident that you cannot perform Maha Bandha for too long.

Do not force yourself; only after several weeks will you be able to perform this Bandha for an entire minute. Note: Nauli Shatkriya's practice will help identify the sphincters involved in the Uddiyana and Mula Bandhas. Pay special attention to the word "identifying": it means bringing into conscious focus some part of your body—external or internal. "Identifying" also implies paying close attention to a sensation produced by internal or external body parts (muscles, organs, or tissues). Feeling hot or cold is one such sensation. Similarly, breathing cold air is all about experiencing the coldness in the passages of your nostrils and windpipe.

Some Minor Bandhas

1. **Hand Lock**: Clenching your fists. If you have practiced martial arts, you know there are two or three ways of curling your fingers and thumb into a tight fist. It is OK if you do not, but you must remember also to clench your little finger. One usually forgets to do that.

2. **Foot Lock**: Curl your toes and keep them clenched tightly. Again, do not forget to clench your little toes.

3. **Face Lock**: Contort your face, clench your teeth and jaw, and press your lips firmly together. This bandha works on different parts of your facial muscles. Smiling involves about 12 muscles, and frowning involves about 11 muscles. (Nine of these 11 frowning muscles differ entirely from the smiling muscles.)

The 5 Fives—Systems of Reality

Tantra offers several systems to comprehend reality, where "Reality" is the composite whole of any experience. Evolution has enabled the human brain to detach itself to create a "mind" separate from the "body." Similarly, reality is an environment in which the observer, the observed, and the things we do not watch are all parts of Reality.

Therefore, in any environment, reality is the entire environment (including you, your thoughts, and your emotions) and the observed and unobserved objects of that environment. You may not notice the flowers when you look at a snake amid a jasmine bush. However, you, the snake, and the flowers are all parts of that reality. Thus, Reality is relative, just like Motion in Physics. When you observe a man walking, the man is moving, but when you are in a moving car, even the roadside tree appears to be moving!

Tantra presents consciousness as one word encapsulating all reality, but our minds break it into its components. We can never focus on all the features of reality; different people will focus on other aspects of that given environment. By understanding these other systems, we can comprehend what truth is.

5 Layers of Self

1. **Environment/Body**

   One exists in this external environment. Though the environmental objects are outside the body, we need to realize how superficial the body's boundary is. Are the clothes I am wearing a part of my body? Is my car my exoskeleton? Anyone who loves their car will understand this notion better. My conscious Self extends to my car to care for it and the space "I" need when driving it.

2. **Mind-Heart**

   The Mind and the Symbolic Heart are a continuum of thought and action or thought and emotion. The Heart we are discussing here is the symbolic representation of feelings and actions. In Tantra, these are not separate because one influences the other, and we need to understand that Mind and Heart are linguistic manifestations of the same entity.

3. **The Life Force**

   Consider this layer: everything in our body that we cannot control: the autonomic nervous system, from the hormones to the blood to our DNA and RNA. Tantra did not discover these entities hundreds of years ago. Still, it was apparent even then that our life force emanates from several bodily systems over which we have no control.

4. **The Void**

   We are now entering a domain where English translations of the descriptive Sanskrit words do not exist or make little sense.

These words are also meaningless because their interpretations vary in different tantric texts. The best way to explain the Void is to compare it to a dreamless sleep. In dreamless sleep, we are not dead; we exist, but there is no "I" and no prefrontal cortex brain activity. We can achieve this state of consciousness through tantric meditation.

Additionally, medical science has shown that this state is comparable to a narcotic-drug-induced high. Tantra warns us about this and even states that the symptoms are not unlike those of a drug addict.

It's, therefore, essential to have a Guru (even if it's on email) while practicing some of these advanced tantric techniques.

5. **Supreme Consciousness**

The absolute layer in Tantra is the Supreme Consciousness: a state of being that ascends indefinitely or descends into the tiny core of existence. This state is the primal source of the Self. It is not local, and I can only describe it as the "energy" that creates its description. I can also compare this to Samadhi; it is erroneous to think we can attain Samadhi only after death.

Samadhi is the ultimate state of Supreme Consciousness—one can experience it and then return to mundane levels of existence. It is this state that Tantric Masters wish to achieve—and return to—when they are ready to die.

5 States of Awareness

In Tantra Yoga, there are four states of awareness depending on how awake or sleepy we are. The fifth state is a state of awareness that needs cultivation: one must practice hard to discover or create it. Of the five states of awareness, we see four through waves of an EEG (electroencephalogram), corresponding to states of wakefulness/sleepiness:

1. **Wakeful State**

    This is the state of awareness when we are awake. Beta waves correspond with this state; these are low-amplitude waves with a high frequency (over 14 cycles per second). We are most excitable in our wakeful state because we are active physically and mentally.

    However, Tantra Masters have called this the least awakened state because we go about our daily chores and everyday life like automatons. Perhaps even like animals who engage only with simple entertainment, food, sleep, and excretion.

    Simply because we are awake and active does not mean we are in the most "aware" state!

2. **Relaxed State**

    When we are not engaged in intense physical or mental activity, we are in a Relaxed State. Alpha waves of the EEG correspond to this state of awareness, and they have frequencies ranging from 8 to 13 cycles per second. Some types of meditation that help you relax and de-stress enable you to reach this state of awareness. I mention only "some types of meditation" because other types can excite you.

3. **The Dream State**

    All these states of awareness are continuous, so you will notice a hypnotic state before entering the dream state. You can experience this if you remind yourself to "look for it" before falling asleep. Your thoughts become nonsensical, and you may hear voices/sounds or feel entirely imaginary sensations but feel real. These sounds/sensations are hypnagogic hallucinations.

Don't worry; these are pretty normal. This is a transitory state between the Relaxed State and the Dream State. Theta waves correspond to this state and have a frequency of 4 to 7 cycles per second. From the frequency, it should be clear that lower frequencies show lower mental activity. This does not mean diminished mental capacity! It implies greater focus and greater concentration.

Some drugs slow mental processes or make us feel like everything is happening slowly. They also heighten our sensory perceptions. With practice, Tantra can help you achieve this state without drugs. Many tantriks today want to accomplish these mental states through shortcuts, so they resort to drugs. Their success is short-lived, and the physical damage caused by drug usage is apparent!

4. **Deep Sleep State**

Delta waves correspond to this state of awareness; they have high amplitudes and frequencies below four cycles per second. This is a state of unawareness in the physical sense and is the diametric opposite of the Wakeful State. This is complete "relaxation" in the genuine sense of the word. There are no dreams; you will achieve this state if you diligently practice Shavasana. Thus, if you want to achieve Delta waves, get a good night's rest!

5. Permeating All Four States

Beyond the Fourth State of Awareness, and simultaneously within each state of awareness, lives the Fifth State. This state does not lie on a scale, but one can say, "… is the scale itself." It makes little sense if you do not experience it, and because it is in the domain of the Occult, it remains indescribable. However, you can comprehend it in the following manner: The mind is twisted, strained, tortured or relaxed, stilled, quieted, calmed… to invent an uncommon state of awareness.

That is how Tantra works! Remember, Tantra comes from two words: tanoti (expand) and trayate (liberate). Expanded consciousness is as infinite as space, so there is no limit to altering or raising one's consciousness. The Fifth State of Awareness and the Zero Level of Tattva are milestones on the tantric journey!

5 Powers of God

A complete realization of the Powers available to human beings is God! Tantra offers us an opportunity to reach the God-Level!

1. Power of Consciousness

In this context, Consciousness is Wakeful Awareness. Many higher-order animals have this power, as they are conscious of themselves. Nevertheless, are they aware of having consciousness? Similarly, simply because a few humans introspect on their consciousness does not mean all humans can do the same.

2. **Power of Bliss**

    This is the ability to know what happiness means and to work towards it. When you think about it, almost all creatures other than humans have this Power in much greater abundance. Compared to other animals, humans come across as nothing more than malcontents do.

3. **Power of Free Will**

    Free will is the power to act upon something or exercise a choice. Tantra offers us this freedom. We continue to debate whether we have Free Will, but Tantra is unequivocal about it: We have the Power of Free Will! This power permeates all other powers. The Freedom to choose (for or against), to act (or not to work), and to express oneself (or remain still/quiet) manifests in the Power of Free Will, giving potency to the other powers.

4. **Power of Knowing**

    Knowledge is the overlap of beliefs and truths. If something is true but so "crazy" that I cannot believe it, it does not become knowledge (at least not for me because I cannot accept that truth). Similarly, if people believe something firmly even though it is false, it does not become knowledge. (People believe in God even though they do not exist.) In the tantric context, the Power of Knowledge is the power to distinguish between a belief, a fact, a lie, and so on.

5. **Power of Action**

    This is self-explanatory: Like all the other powers, it manifests through "action." Every human desire is to express their emotions through action. This power manifests the other powers. There is no point in thinking that power exists if one does not "see" it in action!

5 Acts of God

A complete realization of our actions gives us the potency of the Gods.

1. Self-Expression

Humans can express themselves by writing poetry or making an Origami duck, but Gods do not waste time with such trifles! The Act of self-expression is one of creation but also renovation and evolution. In this act, the tantrik says, "Reality's existence is absolute, but I give it color! The absoluteness of space is indisputable, but—as a God—I personify it, give it meaning, and provide its stupid emptiness with some intelligence!"

"Existence, Knowledge, Infinite is the Brahman!" The universe may have created me, but without me, the Universe is nothing… literally! How do you express yourself?

2. Preservation

Every act of self-expression needs preservation. Meditation can help maintain this state of mind, and deep contemplation can ensure automatic maintenance. However, Mihaly Csikszentmihalyi also recognized this psychological state and termed it "flow."

Will you maintain a mundane and vulgar self-expression or preserve an exalted state of mind?

3. **Destruction**

   Humans worry about how to deal with something that has become boring! But not Gods! Gods destroy them. Shiva is the Lord of Destruction, and many scholars explain this benevolently by stating Shiva destroys something because it is evil. Shiva destroys because destruction is necessary for renewal and revival.

   This is false: Shiva destroys because he can, because he is bored. After all, in his infinite wisdom—destruction is as exciting and entertaining as creation!

   Try not to comprehend this as a human; imagine it as a Tantric God! Additionally, think of death as destruction, and you will arrive at a socially meaningful interpretation of death. It will stop being a phenomenon that requires divine explanation.

4. **Forgetting**

   Have you ever tried to forget something but could not? The undesirable thought or spiteful memory keeps returning no matter how hard you try. Now imagine a power that can make the thought/memory go away as quickly as turning something off. Our brains are profoundly complex and can remember almost everything right from birth (some tantriks say even from inside the womb), but it is also complicated enough to let us quickly forget something. Tantra teaches us how.

5. **Remembering**

   This complements Forgetting, and both these facets of the mind are forms of the expansion and contraction of consciousness.

In a rather simplistic manner, people say that a computer and the brain are similar: each can take in information, store it, and recall specific bits. The brain can store immense amounts of data, but the computer is better at remembering information.

Tantra teaches you to recall information with the same reliability as computers. I can tell myself to wake up at a particular time (say 4 a.m.) and do so consistently (give or take 10 minutes). Regardless of how tired I am or jet-lagged, I can "tell myself" to wake up at a specific time, and I will.

I knew this for a long time, but only recently, three scientists (Jeffrey C. Hall, Michael Rosbash, and Michael W. Young) won the Nobel Prize for discovering the molecular mechanisms of body clocks, also known as circadian rhythms.

5 Veils of Ignorance

These are Action, Knowledge, Desire, Time, and Cause and Effect.

(Please refer to the section on Tattvas for a detailed explanation.)

1. **Action (Tattva Level 7)**

    My interpretation of this tattva is "movement." Tantra does not classify this as intelligence but as a moment of reality that manifests through physical actions or "movements" of the body.

2. **Knowledge (Tattva Level 8)**

    All knowledge is limited! We can never fully know something.

3. **Desire (Tattva Level 9)**

Shaiva Tantra encourages us to indulge our desires! The best way to deal with temptation is to give in to it. The best way to deal with cravings is to surrender. Interestingly, a slogan in many Anonymous Groups is "Surrender to Win."

4. **Time (Tattva Level 10)**

This level deals with our perception of the forward movement of time. However, I can recreate an experience using imaginative visualization and return in time.

5. **Cause and Effect (Tattva Level 11)**

We observe that every action causes a reaction and decide (erroneously) that that action will always drive that reaction! Laws of the physical world don't apply to the human world of emotions!

Special Note: All the Veils of Ignorance are positive forces; we need them to function in the wakeful world. We face many choices daily and must make those choices based on limited information. We also need to make those choices quickly to function in society. None of these levels is harmful—they limit us to ensure our survival, comfort, and protection. For example,

- My action potential may be immense, but I must limit my action per a particular task or event.

- I use the notion of Cause and Effect to manipulate things in daily life, but I ought to know that the idea is erroneous for more profound things.

- My tantrik visualization and imagination can transcend time; time's forward movement does not restrict me.

- Knowledge may have limits, but I do not need all information to make decisions.

- You could misplace your Desire: you may "feel" hungry when thirsty. Yoga teachers tell their students to watch for hunger at meal times because they may have felt thirsty instead. Your body merely sends you a message; it does not use specific words like thirst.

This extends to emotions and beliefs: What is your true motivation behind desiring something (fame, power, and glory) or someone? Is your desire satisfied/satiated after achieving that something?

Mind & Consciousness

Consciousness

There is no consensus on consciousness! No definition is accurate enough, no description is complete, and no explanation is satisfactory. Yet, we use it to make sense of our reality and comprehend our environment. Additionally, thanks to Artificial Intelligence, there is a renewed interest in consciousness among computer scientists, neuroscientists, psychologists, and philosophers.

Tantra does not define consciousness; it expands it.

Self- Consciousness

Some aspects of consciousness—such as self-consciousness—help us identify ourselves. I "kind of know" who I am! Dogs and cats also have this awareness. However, do bacteria have self-awareness? Memory serves as a mechanism to remind us of who we are. It does a pretty good job of telling me who I am, but it isn't enjoyable in other aspects. Even if we store all information perfectly (we do not know if that is the case), recall that memory is inefficient—computers do a much better job.

Practitioners of Tantra can often recall memories from many years ago, which lends credence to the statement that the brain stores all information. Besides memories, Tantra Yoga can also evoke sensations from the past, and many of these can be vividly real. Self-awareness (conscious of being conscious) amazes psychologists and philosophers. An example is how Tantra can help us realize being in a dream. In this manner, tantriks often control their dreams and can thus conjure up exciting dream escapades. Being "awake" in a dream is nothing new, but Tantra helps us manage it.

Subjectivity versus Objectivity

Tantra endows reality with consciousness because of reality's inseparability from our intelligence. The subjective nature of reality often appears more logical and provides a better picture of reality than objectivity. Consider the following example: You observe a stranger on the road. Before that moment, the stranger did not exist, and after you have lost sight of that person, you do not know if that person continues to exist. Objectively, you cannot be sure!

Tantra states we create the world—how we see it and how we want to see it.

Awareness of Self-Awareness

In *Shadows of the Mind*, Roger Penrose separates "consciousness" and "awareness." Without getting too academic, think of an amoeba reacting to its environment, and you will comprehend "awareness." When we reflect upon or analyze that awareness (whether in an amoeba or us), only then does that action become consciousness.

Take that a step further: focus on your thinking. You have suddenly fractionated yourself and become the observer. "You" are now observing "yourself." This is not a subtle exercise. We often perform actions without conscious focus, almost like automatons... almost like amoebae. When you observe all your efforts, you become a tantrik!

Science of Consciousness

Penrose defines the scientific study of consciousness and how we perceive reality in his books. Some books are *Shadows of the Mind*, *The Large, the Small and the Human Mind*, and *The Emperor's New Mind*.

Expansion of Consciousness and Tantra

Our popular understanding of consciousness is wakeful awareness. Whatever we experience while awake is "real." However, any serious exploration of this wakeful state will show many forms of this awareness. We live our lives based on our thoughts during this state of awareness.

Our mental state prejudices reality. Our moods affect our perception of reality. Can we confidently state that a universally accepted (objective) reality exists in that context?

How real is a vivid dream or nightmare? How real is a hero or villain in a movie? How real is our experience of joy or pain? Tantra makes all of reality a part of consciousness by making awareness a part of any instance of reality. Tantra categorizes our distinct realities in the form of different Tattvas.

The 36 Levels of Reality, as revealed in the Shaivism Tattvas, provide us with a deeper and expansive understanding of consciousness.

The Brain

Many believe the brain is the best place to look for evidence of consciousness. If a person is aware of something, the awareness arises in the brain. Many scientists and Penrose assert that there is not insufficient logical evidence for consciousness, so we cannot start using scientific tools to prove it. Any neuroscientist can also make a strong case that consciousness could be several things depending on the brain activity the researcher is recording.

Different activities (when awake and asleep) evoke different brain reactions, so consciousness may differ at different times. This is untenable: possibly, the brain produces consciousness in the same way that it has all other kinds of information and that consciousness exists at the same level as all the additional information.

Consider this: You watch TV while eating but have no taste of the food because you focus entirely on the TV.

The cerebral cortex is the largest site of neural integration in the central nervous system. It plays a crucial role in attention, perception, awareness, thought, memory, language, and consciousness. Therefore, unless the cerebral cortex processes the information of a particular sensation, we will not experience it!

Who am I?

- A person can be in a state of self-awareness and not be aware of it. Example: When you awaken from sleep, you may ask yourself, "Where am I?" but never, "Who am I?" (Unless you are Jason Bourne!)

- You are wide awake, see something on the floor in your house, and know instantly that it is a piece of rope.

- You are drugged or drunk and see something on the floor. You are not sure what it is; you investigate, and depending on your state of intoxication, you will realize it is a rope or imagine it is a snake.

- You are fast asleep, and a cobra slithers across your body. You may not wake up!

In each of the above, your consciousness is fully functional, but your awareness is at different levels. We often confuse 'Consciousness' and 'Awareness' for each other, causing much confusion on the question: What is consciousness?

According to Tantra, everything is consciousness: memory of a piece of music, craving for ice cream, the pain of an ankle sprain, or the happiness of love. Your heart is beating, your lungs are functioning, and your guts are moving the food inside you... you are not aware of it all the time, but you are always conscious. Food on the plate soon becomes a part of you. The outside air gets into your lungs and becomes a part of you. Your dead skin becomes a part of the environment daily. Your clothes are as much a part of you when it is bitterly cold as your car is a part of your body when driving.

The external becomes the internal—breathing and the things we see and touch. The sensations of the external objects reverberate within us—it is all consciousness. If something becomes a part of us, can we not say we have become a part of that thing? If I eat a banana, the banana (because it is smaller) becomes a part of me. However, if I eat an elephant, can I confidently say that I have become a part of the elephant? Have I become the banana? Have I become the elephant?

Cognitive Science

Cognitive Science differs from the Science of Consciousness. The former has made tremendous advances because it concerns itself with understanding and changing behavior based on observations, but the latter is stagnating at the level of wordplay. One example is the phrase "conscious awareness"—as if we need to define something in such hair-splitting detail!

Therefore, while we know (perhaps subconsciously) what consciousness is and is not, we still cannot put a finger on it. We know a moving car is not conscious, and we know a sleeping cat has consciousness, but try isolating the determining factors, and this foxes us completely.

Many scholars take consciousness for granted and try to study it purely from the point of view of observational data: What is present in brain function, and what is absent in brain damage? Brain Science gives us a picture of what the brain can and cannot do. It gives us different forms of awareness wherein we know ourselves—have complete confidence in our identity—and gain knowledge of our environment.

Different brain regions "light up" under different situations, but what light pattern or "photograph" of the neuronal network should we attribute to consciousness? Any neuroscientist would be glad to know if consciousness exists purely inside the brain because scholars have postulated it may not be so.

Tantra explores consciousness by categorizing the psychological and physical interaction into 36 levels of experience: The 36 Tattvas of Shaiva Tantra.

A Billion Plus

When a particular set of neurons or a specific neuronal network (biological neural network) is activated, it evokes a memory. In addition, any new experience creates new synaptic connections. Not all of this is under our control. It happens on its own, the same way the billion-plus nerve cells in the spinal cord react to stimuli, leading to the "reflex action."

Similarly, the cerebellum controls our balance and complex movements when walking or running. We also take our bipedal balance for granted! Damage to the spinal cord or the cerebellum causes several handicaps—from paralysis to not having the original adeptness with the fingers. However, there is not an iota of damage to consciousness. Trauma to the brain can also cause amnesia, but the amnesiac knows himself—as a human being—even if he does not know his name or does not remember some or all of his past. He may have forgotten everything, but his consciousness is intact!

There are over 80 billion neurons in the brain, and somehow, the mechanism of consciousness processes information as a mere serial processor—one bit of data at a time. Albeit, it does this rapidly, so we get the impression of managing many things simultaneously.

The Cerebral Cortex

Because the cerebral cortex gives us much of our logic and awareness to deal with the physical world, we desperately desire to have consciousness "live" there. Sadly, consciousness does not make this brain region its exclusive domain. Epileptic patients with *grand mal* seizures often have parts of the brain removed to prevent the onset of a seizure or to prevent the seizure from spreading to the other parts of the brain.

When surgeons removed tissue from the prefrontal cortex, consciousness had no impact. However, when surgeons excised parts of the posterior cortex, the patients could not recognize faces or identify a color. These are essential aspects of consciousness, but not all of it, and evidently, the patients slowly learned to compensate for their loss. One such patient shook his head vigorously to respond to test questions. It was almost as if he was making neuronal connections by shaking his head.

Subjective experience also posits consciousness in other parts of the brain or other parts of the body. Feeling something in the heart or having a gut feeling may be literal experiences! Brain damage may or may not lead to vegetative states, and even in a vegetative state, the person may be conscious but unable to communicate. However, if we do not know what consciousness is, how can one identify its presence or absence in abnormal situations?

The Conscious Space

Tantra classifies consciousness as the entire space within which an experience occurs. Experience presumes intelligence, and intelligence presumes life. We won't discuss defining intelligence or life, but let it suffice that we recognize both qualities. At least, most of us do not speak to lampposts!

By expanding—consciousness, Tantra takes even life and intelligence out of the creature and into the conscious space of experience. Consciousness constantly expands and contracts; when we realize this, we can learn techniques to expand and contract our consciousness at will. Research has also shown that a small set of neural networks cannot create consciousness—we need something massive and interconnected.

By interconnecting billions of neurons capable of forming new connections, we get a hypothesis for consciousness creation.

36 Tattvas

Shaivism's 36 Tattvas: What Reality Is!

What is a Tattva? There is no literal translation of the word "tattva." Superficially, one can say that a tattva is a thing or an attribute or intelligence. In that context, it is a thing, quality, *and* intelligence combined. You will understand as you read further, but for now, accept that a tattva is a consciousness: when we explore each one, you will see how even a thing can gain "intelligence."

Traditional Yoga propounded the tattvas, but Shaiva Tantra Yoga introduced several additional tattvas, taking the number to 36. We describe these 36 Tattvas as levels of reality. It is only for convenience's sake that we speak of "Levels of Reality" because many of these tattvas seemingly manifest "outside of ourselves."

In Shaiva Tantra, this is a delusion, but we need to isolate the tattvas to understand them. Therefore, the external tattvas represent the most superficial levels of reality, and—as we go higher in the hierarchy—the tattvas represent more profound levels of reality.

Here, I present the 36 Tattvas of Shaivism, from the lower to higher/deeper:

Level 36 to Level 32: Earth, Water, Fire, Wind, Space

In tantric traditions, the five essential elements of nature are the first and most apparent levels of reality. One realizes the tattvas are not only "levels" of reality but also different "forms" of reality because you really cannot say that Earth is the lowest level, so it is less critical than Wind or Fire.

To understand why these are also attributes, one has to perceive these elements with their associated characteristics: Wind for breezy, cold, forceful, etc.; Fire for heat, burning, energy, etc.; Water for cold, wet, flowing, etc.; and so on.

It is also evident that these do not exist individually, and we find them in varying combinations. For example, each tattva occupies Space, and Space as a tattva exists within each–even within an atom!

Level 31 to Level 27: Odor, Flavor, Appearance, Touch, Sound

In Tantra, everything has these characteristics to a greater or lesser degree. Consider a menu item in a fancy restaurant: besides ensuring it tastes excellent, the chef puts considerable effort into making the plate look artistic. Where is the sound? It's in the ambient music!

This is an excellent example to understand how the "tattva of the dish" does not "live" merely within the confines of the dish. Similarly, a tattva—any tattva—can manifest outside the confines of the space the object is occupying and outside of the one primary/striking attribute it possesses.

Level 26 to Level 22: Intestines (for expelling), Genitals (for reproducing), Feet (for locomotion), Hands (for holding), Mouth (for chewing/talking)

We experience many realities only through the instruments with which we access them. We may not understand the existence of a thing without touching it, and—to touch something—we may need to hold it. Holding that thing will also give us an idea of how firm or flexible, wet or dry, or hot or cold it is. Only when our Hands reach out to hold something do we "touch" it!

We may control our Hands, Feet, and Mouth, but we do not control our Intestines and Genitals. The autonomic nervous system controls the latter two.

Level 21 to Level 17: Nose, Tongue, Eyes, Skin, Ears

The sense organs are our direct contact with reality. In Tantra, these are the gateways to the spiritual path for every tantric practitioner, and many cleansing rituals exist to ensure that we keep these tattvas healthy. Each sense organ gives us a distinct sense of reality that may or may not be better! Dogs have about 300 million olfactory receptors compared to about 6 million human receptors. Does this mean that a dog's sense of olfactory reality is so many times superior? Yes, and it additionally implies a unique sense of reality.

Qualia

"The status of qualia is hotly debated in philosophy, largely because it is central to a proper understanding of the nature of consciousness. Qualia are at the very heart of the mind-body problem." Plato Project, Stanford University

A quale (singular of qualia) is a person's subjective experience. It is an intrinsic sensation one feels, knows, and usually does not put into words. One may put it into words only to get a grasp of it because language provides us with words to "grasp" the meaning of something. In doing so, we "give" meaning to things but reduce our unique experiences to the lowest common denominator of a common language.

If we had words for ourselves—a personal and private language—then there would be no problem. However, Ludwig Wittgenstein has already shown how a private language is impossible. Hence, Tantra provides us with techniques to communicate with ourselves using symbols and sounds that appeal to our inner cognitive workings. These systems of mantras and mandalas bypass the vocabulary and syntax of languages.

Tantra also tells us that specific, ritualized actions can bypass the vulgar (commonplace, lacking sophistication) communication systems.

Thus, Tantra prioritizes the importance of action to experience a more profound reality.

The Sensual World

Tantra stresses exploiting the sensual world for its own sake. Education has stunted our Five Senses, so meditative indulgences of these senses are necessary to complete our Self. However, we have taken this as a license for all luxuries, leading to addiction and corruption. One such example is tantric sex. Tantric sex is not merely about sexual acts but sexual meditation. It teaches diversity in love—not a variety of lovers.

Warning: *If you cannot draw the line between meditative "tasting" and licentious indulgence, do not start. Once addiction sets in, you may not even realize it, denying your addiction until it ends in insanity, imprisonment (in a jail or mental institution), or death! In Alcoholics Anonymous (and practically every Anonymous group), there is a common refrain: "The idea that somehow, someday, he will control and enjoy his drinking is the great obsession of every abnormal drinker. The persistence of this illusion is astonishing. Many pursue it to the gates of insanity or death."*

Level 16 to Level 12: Mind, Ego, Intelligence, Instinct, Consciousness

It is essential to mention that Yoga—besides the practice of physical exercises—also includes training the mind. Specific asanas (yogic postures or poses) in many Yoga Schools enhance particular attitudes. One yoga asana may teach us humility, while another yoga posture may teach us devotion.

16. Mind

This is one's ability to pay attention. Focusing your mind, paying attention, concentrating on a task, etc., is at the level of the mind.

15. Ego

This is one's ability to create an idea of the Self and form an image of the Self (a picture of one's personality). I create the impression of Myself! However, the Ego diminishes when we grow older. Unlike most people, a self-centered person has a small ego, so they behave in a manner wherein they have to protect what little they have.

In contrast, a child has a massive ego because it possesses everything it sees or perceives.

The infant sees itself in everything! Everything is within the sphere of itself! The infant has no sense of material possession, so its consciousness is posited in every object or creature it perceives. A doll or a warm blanket is as living as a parent is. A pet cat or dog is identical to itself.

However, as the infant grows, its experiences limit and constrain the Self. Fire is painful, a beetle is bitter, and mud is distasteful… these unpleasant experiences are imprinted and lead the child to form the notion of "Not Me" or a "painful/unpleasant" thing. Adding to the "Not Me" list, the idea of "Me" gets refined and limited.

In the modern world—especially in Western, industrialized societies—ego often creates the most significant barrier to self-realization.

An Egotist is arrogant, boastful, self-centered, and selfish, while an Egoist is only self-centered and selfish. Either way, the Shaivism Tattvas allows everyone to become the Supreme Ego!

14. Intelligence

This is the popular understanding of "intelligence." When the "Me" starts separating from the "Not Me," a mental mechanism must create the distinction. Intelligence does this by enabling differentiation between things. Thanks to Howard Gardner, we know of 8 (probably even 9) distinct intelligences, each having origins in the brain.

Mind & Consciousness

Psychologists and educationists suspected these separate intelligences, but it was only after Gardner (*Frames of Mind*) confirmed it we realized these different intelligences.

13. Instinct

Instincts are perhaps the most noticeable aspects of our consciousness. If one ignores them, they remind you by slapping you in the face. Here is an instinct that you may not be familiar with even kids who are born blind will smile when happy. Smiling is an instinct; smile more!

12. Consciousness

In most Yoga Systems, this is the highest form of "experience," but not in Shaiva Tantra. A simple form of Tantra meditation will reveal the many diverse manifestations of this tattva. Consciousness is that framework within which the other tattvas exist. Reality requires the platform of consciousness to manifest itself, and consciousness is the vessel that holds reality.

You may ask, "What about the reality outside the vessel?" Then consciousness will expand and engulf that, too. Therefore, if you think about the Earth, then the Earth manifests within your consciousness; the minute you think of the moon, the moon is also engulfed. Please move to the galaxy, and consciousness expands to include it.

Thus, your consciousness is unlimited. Jean Paul Sartre describes this behavior of consciousness as "ever over-flowing." In astronomical space, the farther we travel, the deeper we go into our minds.

Level 11 to Level 7: Cause and Effect, Time, Desire, Knowledge, Action *(Also known as the 5 Veils of Ignorance)*

Level 11: Cause and Effect

Intelligence helps us distinguish between objects and processes. It concludes its observations. It sees action and the effect of that action and makes universal statements about the same. It seems every action has a reaction and decides that that action will always cause that reaction! So we all know about "cause and effect," and our lives run on it. However, we never stop thinking about a particular action's cause.

If I light a match and take it to firewood (action), the wood will catch fire (reaction). Going deeper, why can't I consider the lighting of the match as a reaction? What was the cause? Why did I light the matchstick? OK! I was feeling cold. Why was I feeling cold? Because it is cold outside? Why is it cold outside? Because it is winter? And so on…

The entire business of cause and effect crumbles because of this endless regression into causality. However, it is vital for navigation through our daily lives!

Level 10: Time

To be precise, this level deals with our perception of the forward movement of time. We say it rained for an hour if it rains from 3 pm to 4 pm. We cannot travel back in time, except, of course, in Science Fiction! This is the forward march of time, and we are its slaves. However, every reality experience is subject to how advanced the human being is. With visualization, I can recreate the experience and go back in time.

If I have practiced enough tantric meditation, I can even "feel" the sensations of the past event! No empirical parameters fix an event in time; nothing stops me from returning to that experience. Time moves forward, but my subjective experience can travel in any direction! When tantriks say they can travel in time, they mean (because of visualization and vivid imagination techniques) that the experience is as real as when they had in the past.

Some literature even states that the experience is "more real" because it is bereft of the external physical environment, which dilutes the stimulus.

Level 9: Desire

The strongest desire expressed is the intimacy of sex. This does not need any explanation, but here is a fresh perspective: Most spirituality is ascetic. I remember someone telling me that spiritual awakening is possible only through chastity and poverty! I thought he was joking when he first said it because it sounded like a good joke.

Shaiva Tantra encourages you to dump this kind of crap! Desire—especially sexual intimacy—is natural for any higher-order creature; ignoring or negating it only leads to psychological conditions.

We should indulge our desires! Elaborate tantric rituals exist for the sex act and even for foreplay. Using sex within the context of tantric practice leads to existential satisfaction and even existential healing.

Level 8: Knowledge

In Tantra, all knowledge is limited! When you realize knowledge is nothing but the overlap of beliefs and truths, then all personal knowledge is a matter of convenience. It does not reflect reality from the perspective of objectivity, nor does it alleviate the trained subjective mind of the tantrik.

Only an idiot knows everything; a wise man knows how much he does not know… which is quite a lot!

Level 7: Action

My interpretation of this tattva is "movement." According to Howard Gardner, we have 8 or 9 different intelligences. Bodily-kinesthetic intelligence is one of these 8 or 9 intelligences, and sports people, dancers, and others like them have cultivated it to a great extent. All humans have this intelligence to greater or lesser degrees. Tantra does not classify this as intelligence but as a moment of reality that manifests through physical actions or "movements" of the body.

The Occult Tattvas

Level 6 to Level 0 Maya, Wisdom, God, Beyond God, Shakti, Shiva, The Secret Tattva

Tantric Occult Science explores Tantra in the modern context. However, to understand the unique attributes of Tantric Occultism, we must first understand Occultism itself. Occultism is the domain of human consciousness that one cannot express in words. Every human being has emotions that are similar but not identical. (*Refer to the section on Qualia.*) In this context, Occult experiences are not daily occurrences.

Level 6: Maya

Maya is an illusion, and illusion is everything! Therefore, everything is Maya! In Tantric Occult Science, these statements are genuine.

Remember that we are questioning 'Reality' and challenging the popular idea of 'Reality.' We need to interpret "illusion" as "illumination." Light falls on an object, and we can see it—that is Maya. Neurons fire and thoughts emerge in the brain: that too is Maya.

Maya is everything that manifests itself either as an object or as a thought. The power of appearance (thing or thought) is Maya. Maya is imagination in its totality: from the 'image' of an object the eye creates in the brain to fantasies to conjuring thoughts.

Level 5: Wisdom

Level-Five Wisdom is wisdom in its classical sense: a vibration every creature possesses. A smell, a sound, a rhythm, a color… anything that "vibrates" within us and connects us to our environment purely through non-verbal means is wisdom. The wind is blowing, and the trees are swaying in its flow. The wind is also rustling my hair as if they are leaves. It is raising the dust and the pollen and making crows and butterflies dance in the air: this is wisdom.

Wisdom is the non-verbal realization arising out of our minds' framework. It is not smartness but an innate form of consciousness that everyone is born with. Howard Gardner (Multiple Intelligences Theory) has alluded to a Ninth Intelligence called Existential Intelligence (asking deep questions about life, questioning spirituality, metaphysical intelligence). I believe that Wisdom and Existential Intelligence fall in the same category.

Level 4: God

This is the standard concept of God. Tantra states that everyone has a personal deity (call it what you may or may not name it), which is the level on which we place all known gods. This level of consciousness does not separate itself from anything else. This consciousness sees itself in everything (omnipresence) and can identify the other as itself.

"I am that; that am I!"

God is each individual's personal and private affair, so there are as many gods as the people with a belief system. Even if you believe in 'One God,' your idea of that one god is always unique. Therefore, Tantra states that there are many gods, even if you call them by one name or many names or prefer not to name them at all!

This level is not the prerogative of some unknown (or unknowable) supernatural being—anyone can attain it. It is also unsurprising to see cats, snakes, and other animals worshiped as gods. In animism, nature and animals gain the stature of a god. Thus, you can be God and then go beyond God!

Level 3: Beyond God

The formative principles of a fully expanded mind will naturally lead to realizing a consciousness beyond the ultimate. When a tantrik attains the god level, it soon bores him.

They will create—or become the causative agent—for an idea that exceeds god. Many people continue to use the word "God" for levels of consciousness beyond this, but not an atheist like me.

If God is at the level of milk chocolate, then dark chocolate is beyond god. Different percentages of dark chocolate will make up different levels beyond plain milk chocolate! For the Master, this can happen with each percentage point, but let us consider 55% dark, 80% dark, and 95% dark chocolates, and you will know what I am talking about.

If you still do not get it, try these dark chocolates, and you will learn this truth.

Level 2 and Level 1: Shakti and Shiva

Shakti and Shiva are not deities as popularly worshiped. Tantric Occult Science states that deep levels of consciousness exist simultaneously but are experienced sequentially. Shakti is the creative force: we experience Shakti as the constant flow of thoughts, and Shiva is the space of stillness between the views. Shiva is subtle, and Shakti is evident and in your face.

One attains Shakti, but one can only achieve Shiva. The feminine and masculine forms are for linguistic convenience and make no difference to the ideas of Shiva and Shakti. Any association with feminine and masculine virtues is inconsequential. One could call Shakti masculine and Shiva feminine, which would make no difference in Tantra. (Some schools of Tantra consider Shiva feminine and Shakti masculine.)

You can experience Shakti and Shiva by practicing some Pranayama (breathing exercises). The inhaling and exhaling are Shakti, and holding your breath between these acts is Shiva. In meditation, it is the experience of stillness between the flows of thoughts: the silence of time between one thought leaving and another entering.

There are many techniques to experience these levels of consciousness, but Shiva and Shakti are not explainable or describable—you have to "feel" them. Consider this exercise from a

Buddhist practice: take a sip of water and hold it in your mouth. Do not fill your mouth. Now, depending on how you expand or contract your cheeks, you will "feel" your mouth full of water or air.

Similarly, when doing Pranayam, instead of focusing on the air coming in and going out of your lungs, focus on the emptiness of the lungs filling up (while inhaling) and then the lungs becoming empty again (while exhaling). The breathing exercise has not changed, but your mind now focuses on the emptiness rather than the air coming and going.

Another example: We enjoy a full stomach, especially when the food is good, but try enjoying an empty stomach. I am not talking about starving, but simple fasting: the experience of the space within our body can be pretty exciting. This emptiness is Shiva!

Level 0: The Secret Tattva

This tattva is a secret because one tantrik's experience of it differs from that of another tantrik. This is at the highest level of tattvas because it encompasses all the other tattvas, including Shakti and Shiva. It is the level of the pure Occult—no words can describe the experience. Words will be a waste of paper, and reading those words will be a waste of time.

Essentially, this is a secret not because we keep it that way but because my experience is unique, indescribable, and incomprehensible to another Yogi.

Tantra Meditation

I learned to meditate when I was four years old. At that age, meditation was nothing more than being able to sit still for a few minutes, say about 15-20 minutes. It was an excellent task for a four-year-old, and I am proud to say I accomplished it. Here, I provide my perspective and experience of meditation since then.

What is meditation?

Anyone with the slightest inkling of meditation knows that meditation has many benefits. Sitting quietly and focusing on your breath relaxes, and I will not argue about whether you consider this meditation. However, there are two types of meditation: focused and unfocused. Within these two categories lie all the different meditation techniques.

Some forms of meditation are relaxing, others exhilarating, and others transcendental. Whichever form you attain through any specific technique, all meditation is transformational. It transforms your consciousness and your awareness. In this context, you need to understand consciousness to achieve tremendous success with meditation.

However, "What is meditation?" A state in which you focus your consciousness on something other than the mundane is meditation. You can practice meditation in any posture: sitting, standing, or lying down. You can do it in noisy, busy, or quiet environments. Additionally, you can do it morning or evening, happy or sad, angry or loving, bored or excited... you get the idea.

T'ai Chi is "meditation in motion," the highest form of meditation in Tantra is when you meditate while in movement. Therefore, when you ask, "What is meditation?" the following three states are vital:

1. **Be Aware**: You need to be aware of your surroundings or the machinations of your thoughts. This information need not come from your wakeful consciousness alone—your autonomic nervous system will do most of the work. Your body will tell you how to make yourself comfortable, but you must be in a posture that will not make you fall asleep.

2. **Be Conscious**: I want to distinguish between awareness and consciousness. While awareness is a living body's interaction with its environment, consciousness is about being self-aware. Example: While eating, one can say, "The mouth is chewing the food." One is aware of the chewing, but in meditative consciousness, the statement would be, "'I' am eating, and 'my' mouth is chewing the food." It is essential to be self-aware/conscious of your actions and deliberately connect the self to the activity.

3. **Be In Control**: While unfocused meditation expects that you do not control your thoughts, you still need to flit from focusing on your ideas to not concentrate on them. Example: A thought enters your mind, and you are engaged with it. After a while, you must disengage from that thought and let it go. This is easier said than done! However, if you practice Step 2 above, you will achieve Step 3 quickly.

Forms of Meditation: Active and Passive

Active meditation happens when you perform everyday tasks, stroll, talk, eat, and so on—but you must do all these things consciously and wholly immersed in your studies! This is the aim of Yoga, permitting you to meditate while taking part in worldly pursuits.

Passive meditation is when you sit in one position and allow the subconscious mind to take over. Both forms of meditation go through the following phases:

1. *Preparation*

2. *Relaxation*

3. *Intensification*

4. *Effortless Meditation*

When effortless meditation begins, limitless knowledge and energy manifest themselves. This is the "sensation" of infinity and immortality. Regular practice leads to attaining the state quickly, and eventually, there is no distinction between contrived practice and daily life activities. At this stage, passive meditation becomes unnecessary, and one achieves self-realization. The individual lives totally according to the innermost feelings that— for lack of a proper vocabulary—we call divine.

These emotions have nothing to do with religion or God! The self-realized person can live both a spiritual (as defined by the person himself) and a material existence with no conflict. There is no duality between the two because there is a spontaneous and continuous experience of active meditation. Individuals identify completely with products of perception, even the worldly ones.

Benefits of Meditation

Relaxation is not the only goal of meditation—it is simply a superficial benefit. Most meditative practices focus on concentration and transcendence. It is also a misconception that this can occur only after years of practice. You can achieve the benefits of meditation within a few months, if not within a few weeks.

It is essential to practice the Yoga asanas and pranayamas to prepare the body for meditation and maintain the benefits of meditation; one must continue the practices and intensify them.

Tantric Meditation Techniques

Most basic forms of meditation ask you to focus on your breath. This is a great place to start: it is the most fundamental physical activity that the autonomic nervous system controls. Yet we can exert some control over it by breathing slowly/rapidly or deeply/superficially. This form of meditation is great for beginners because you can engage in focused or unfocused meditation with this technique. In focused meditation, you can control your breathing; in unfocused meditation, you "observe" your breathing, helping you maintain minimal control.

Tantric meditation techniques are unique in the sense that they offer simple but powerful tips. One example is using the "observation" technique in everyday tasks/emotions. Through pranayama, we can associate breathing with every emotion or activity. Therefore, we are meditating on how our breath changes with different emotions or observing the effect of other physical activities on our breath.

Be aware of these simple steps, practice them, and you will expand or contract your mind through meditation. You will become as big as a mountain or as small as a muon (an elementary particle similar to

Mind & Consciousness

the electron but with much greater mass). You need not be skeptical! Our consciousness does not exist in any fixed part of the body, nor does an external limit bind it. Our adult brain imposes limitations on our consciousness.

Through any focused thought process (you may not want to call it meditation), your consciousness can descend into the tiny or ascend to the infinite. Too much?! Consider the following situations:

- Our suspension of disbelief when we watch a movie: How immersed are we? To what extent do we identify/become the principal character/protagonist of the film?

- Recently, a virtual reality software program recreated a woman's dead child. Moved to tears, the mother reached out and 'touched' the 3D version of her child. To what extent did the mother consider her child real?

- Research has shown that parts of our brains that fire up (under MRI scanners) during a dream are the same that light up when we're awake. How real are our dreams?

Tantra has documented techniques in meditation to help us create (or recreate) experiences. It tells us how flexible our consciousness can be, how intangible reality is, and how we can exert our will and control over the universe.

Buddhist Meditation

Tantric meditation and Buddhist meditation are similar; historically, the latter is the evolution of genuine Tantra. Buddhist meditation (also meditation within Tibetan Buddhism) is not a religion, but the spiritual tenets of Buddhism do inspire it.

The core of this spirituality is Dhamma (another term for Dharma or the Righteous Path). It is also the most misunderstood concept in many religions, and that is because Dharma is not a religion at all! The righteous path is just that—righteous. It has its internal logic and mechanism and does not require a God to enforce it.

The Four Noble Truths

To sit and contemplate an idea or an object is the act of meditation. If no peace is possible in the world, then at least let us try to find inner peace. This is the basic premise of the Four Noble Truths of Buddhism:

1. Dukkha (pain) arises from physical trauma, emotional problems, and grief.

2. This dukkha is the consequence of desire and obsessions.

3. It is possible to resolve dukkha.

4. There are methods and techniques to resolve dukkha.

Pain is in our genes! We have inherited it from the Neanderthals. However, while we can't get it out of our genes, we can at least deal with the symptoms—especially the psychological ones. The fourth Noble Truth uses meditation as a method or discipline to release people from the bondage of negative feelings. If the primary cause of everyone's agony were psychological, then logic would tell us that the cure, too, could be psychological.

Thus, Buddhism designed mental exercises aimed at easing these psychological problems. Some view meditation as a higher state of the pious life and a step towards sainthood or being holy. Meditation is not an act of converting a sinner to having a more profound commitment to his religion, but a means to achieve serenity. Meditation is a Tantra—merely a technique, but when used within the context of Dharma, it leads to higher consciousness. The goals of this meditation technique differ little from the other methods: they get rid of the Dukkha and attempt to attain Samadhi.

Insight Meditation

Meditation is a method through which an individual gains insight into cosmic knowledge and realizes that bliss is attainable. It plays a part in practically all faiths, although some do not use the word 'meditation' to describe their contemplative practice. Additionally, meditation does not constantly have a spiritual component. It is a natural part of the human experience and helps as a treatment for promoting health and improving the body's immune system.

In Buddhism, the individual meditating is not always trying to get into a hypnotic state, nor are they trying to become a saint! All meditation aims to become 'Chaitanya' or 'The Enlightened.'

When Siddhartha attained Chaitanya, he became Buddha!

Mind-Body

Meditation involves the body and the inner workings of the mind. All guided meditation has the supreme goal of putting an end to duality. This is also the goal of Non-Dual Shaiva Tantra. It is not surprising to see how Buddhism took the principles of Tantra and further refined them. That is why Buddhism and Tantra fascinate us even after 2500 years.

The mind-body experience extends to meditating in a group—maybe at a retreat or among fellow enthusiasts. It shows that we are part of a larger ecosystem involving all creatures.

Dealing with the Mind

We are an accumulation of thoughts that we consciously cultivate or unconsciously imbibe. We perceive the world from our dreary or cheerful disposition in this context. Buddhist Meditation attempts to turn one's awareness away from the world of activity that preoccupies us and leads us to the inner experience of ideas, sensations, and thoughts.

In the Buddhist Tradition, meditation involves achieving balance—a balance between all the tattvas that one is experiencing. These may be the Physical Tattvas or the Occult Tattvas, and the idea is to create harmony between the tattvas.

Methods of Meditation

Some classical meditation techniques use one's breathing. This is the practice of Pranayama within meditation, wherein you concentrate on the breath and its flow. You can even imagine its effects on different parts of the body and other thoughts within your mind. Multitudes of combinations arise when you mix these factors. It is essential to think of the breathing, the person doing the breathing, and the observer observing all this.

This is the essence of tantric meditation: all these entities are the same person, but fractionation of the personality is necessary before we put them together as The Supreme Non-Dual personality or Shiva (The Blessed One). In Buddhism, Buddha replaces Shiva.

Motion and Stillness

The novice will need to use many techniques for meditation: count breaths, focus on a candle, gaze upon a flower, and so on... S/he may also want to sit still in a quiet place, play music, use telling beads and whirling prayer wheels, etc. However, advanced meditation is meditation in motion (walking meditation)—going for a walk, swimming, cleaning the house or garden, serving people in a soup kitchen, walking the dog...

Motion is also manifest in service: "Serving other Creatures" is an essential motto of Buddhist practice. Less advanced religions interpret this narrowly, changing the phrase to "Serving other humans!"

The Trinity of Buddhist Meditation

When a Zen Buddhist (one school of Buddhism) practices meditation, three critical factors come into play:

1. *Motives and Principles*: Are your motives righteous (Dharma) and beneficial to all?

2. *Meditation (Samadhi):* Techniques to turn your gaze inwards and ponder whether the disturbance and Dukkha you see in the world is a projection of your inner self. Is existential emptiness a modern-age phenomenon? Alternatively, is it an aspect of what Howard Gardner calls Philosophical Intelligence?

3. *Penance*: This is not about torturing oneself but involving oneself in acquiring knowledge and pursuing Truth. While engaged in deep study, one has to sacrifice superficial things, which is why it is called penance.

Types of Meditation

There are as many types of meditation—as many as the creatures that are living. However, for convenience, we classify them into five types:

1. *Concentration*: Continuous focus on one object, thought, or emotion. In Buddhism, meditation involves the visualization of complex images of Buddha. This form of meditation can lead you into deeper and deeper states of absorption, known as Dhyana.

2. *Creation*: Creation/Recreation of thoughts, ideas, images, emotions, feelings, memories... Creating happiness through fantasies is a great way to meditate and a significant part of Vama Marga (Left-Hand Path of Tantra) and Tantric Sex.

3. *Sensitization*: Recreating memories from the perspective of senses: taste, smell, touch, and feeling. On a higher level, one sits calmly, aware of what is happening in the environment or the world without judging, fantasizing, or trying to change things. Compassion meditation (developing loving-kindness) is one such example.

4. *Introspection*: Analyses of higher-order thoughts, ideas, and concepts. It also implies paying attention to a theme and being open to whatever arises from the experience.

5. *Reflection*: Thinking of how you analyze and react to your thoughts from the perspective of your sub-personalities. Example: When you watch an exciting movie or read a fascinating book, do you identify with the protagonist at one

point and the antagonist at another? Meditation is not merely idle postures; it involves mindfulness practice in daily life.

Anyone who has practiced Yoga asanas and some meditation will realize how mindfulness practice within mundane activities gives one the "sensation of eternity"—one becomes immortal!

Preparation and Posture

The classical posture is padmasana. If you cannot do the padmasana, try the ardha-padmasana or vajrasana. If that is not possible, you can meditate in any posture so long as you are comfortable, your spine is straight, and you are not likely to fall asleep. Taking time before and after you meditate is helpful to settle into and emerge from the practice.

It is also a good idea to warm up, do some Yoga asanas, and do some breathing exercises (pranayama) before you meditate. Modern medicine increasingly uses meditation and mindfulness in healthcare, especially chronic illnesses and depression. In its Buddhist context, meditation is vital to spiritual awakening. However, learning to meditate is not about following a recipe—you must practice the following before you start:

- Do warm-up exercises before you start your Yoga
- Do your Yoga asanas before doing pranayama
- Do your pranayama before meditation

You can see from the above that each is a complex system we must practice before attempting meditation. The general advice from

Buddhist monks is that it helps to meditate with others and to have a teacher who can help you with issues that arise along the way.

Zen Meditation (Mindfulness Meditation)

This form is about mindfulness because Zen is about living in the present with complete awareness. It is almost like asking, "What am I doing? And why am I doing it?" for every activity—however insignificant—daily. You practice being aware of everything you see, hear, feel, taste, and smell. So when you eat, eat! Don't talk, or read, or watch TV.

Zen practice is to realize that thoughts are a natural faculty of the mind, and we should not stop, ignore, or reject them. It also provides liberation from the anxieties and fears of the morrow that destroy the present! In Zen Buddhism, the purpose of meditation is to stop the mind from rushing about in an aimless (or obsessive/purposeful) stream of thoughts. The aim is "to still the mind."

Meditation, Consciousness, and the Mind

People think they know meditation because they have seen some images of someone sitting quietly with their eyes closed. Meditation is much more! Do animals meditate? If you look at cats, one can only answer in the affirmative! I suspect the same about owls, eagles, snakes, and alligators!

Let us look at the human brain to see how the experience of meditation affects it. We know the mind is conscious, subconscious, and unconscious. These are states of awareness corresponding to wakefulness, sleep, and sleep. Though not entirely correct, they help our popular understanding of the mind.

This is NOT consciousness! Our awareness can also be unconscious, as in the body adapting to slight changes in temperature without us knowing about it. Only when the stimulus becomes extreme does it enter our thinking in the wakeful state. Does the same happen when we are in deep sleep? The temperature drops and makes us pull the blanket closer to us. We are not at all awake, but the body responds.

Mindfulness meditation disregards widespread and erroneous constructs of consciousness and focuses on the fact that consciousness is ever-present in its ultimately potent form, but our awareness is incomplete. Thus, mindfulness helps expand our attention until it achieves the fullness and completeness of consciousness. In this context, phrases such as "higher consciousness," "pure consciousnesses," and "cosmic consciousness" are also entirely erroneous! They should instead be "higher awareness," "pure awareness," and "cosmic awareness!"

Consciousness does not require a prefix or a suffix! Things like inspiration, inner peace, happiness, and transcendental experiences are forms of one or the other awareness. This awareness can also make us go deeper into the background of knowledge, and this is like gaining deeper or unique insights when you read a delightful book repeatedly. It is from this domain that geniuses get their flashes of imagination. It is the source of much more profound knowledge.

Can we think of untiring study as guided meditation? Persistent labor as meditation in motion? Dance as trance? We can, and these forms of meditation are not only mindful but also involve full-body participation.

The Unconscious

Another part of this mind is the cumulative unconscious that Carl Jung did much to extrapolate. This part of the brain has blueprints of the evolutionary past, archetypes, and automatic responses. It links us to all other people because it is the standard template of humankind.

Essentially, it even links us to other primates and mammals! Consider the simian grasp, fear of reptiles, and the smile, and you will comprehend the similarities. Consider also how human societies reflect animal societies; the comprehension is complete. Thus, within these various brain locations is the sensation of consciousness that we call 'Self.'

The Self is consciousness—there is no separation! Tantra states consciousness is the mechanism by which the universe becomes a part of the Self. We cannot understand this logically, but we can experience it in the domain of the Occult when we go into deep meditation.

Meditation aims to achieve calmness (in the preliminary stages) and a higher state of emotion or feeling. We can achieve this through deep meditation or meditation in the subconscious (such as lucid dreaming).

Even if we presume that the center of our being is the ego, a well-nourished ego will illuminate The Self, making us aware of something beyond.

Becoming Gods

What happens when we meditate? When we meditate, we can take our awareness to the various elements of our thoughts. Typically, superficial activities of daily life consume our awareness, but meditation makes us look at ourselves dispassionately, reveals our dark secrets, and unveils deep-rooted complexes. We recognize fears that we were not mindful of earlier.

Before, we were only mindful of the symptoms of worries in the form of anger, hatred, anxiety, etc. When we face these deep-rooted complexes, we can remove them and enjoy life. You will become quite familiar with the internal procedures of your body during meditation because your awareness will extend to the mechanisms that control these bodily functions in the waking state.

In higher states of meditation, consciousness moves to the higher mind or the region operating in the domain of the Occult. Awareness increases beyond rational concepts and often beyond words and language. The goal of meditation is self-realization. People often interpret this as "finding one's true self" as if The Self hides somewhere in our psyche!

In reality, it is the creation of The Self. This is the power of Tantra when it reveals such secrets to us. Don't bother with finding yourself; create a new, gorgeous Self!

Consciousness renders the exploration of the brain and identifies with the fundamental core of an individual's present moment—pure awareness. When someone attains self-realization, it suggests he has contacted his whole being and now recognizes his presence and his life from the viewpoint of the Self and not from someone else's perspective.

In this context, education, indoctrination, and socio-cultural norms become redundant. Not only can we become superhumans, but also Gods!

Raja Yoga (Patanjali's Yoga Sutras): The Eightfold Path

By Ajita Diamond Sinha Lyngdoh

- Yoga sits in the sun, soaking in the warmth and life-giving energy.

- Yoga is watching the rain and listening to its tip-tapping on the leaves and rooftops.

- Yoga is singing, dancing, working, walking, running, playing, laughing, eating…

Patanjali's Yoga Sutras (also called Raja Yoga or the Eightfold Path) can present many challenges; the first one is probably a lack of flexibility, and it is pretty apparent that the goal of Yoga is to achieve physical flexibility. However, Patanjali's Yoga Sutras aim at physical flexibility—the ability to contort one's body in many directions—and mental, emotional, and spiritual flexibility.

What is Spiritual Flexibility?

I was born into a family of mixed cultures. My mother was of Pnar-Khasi parentage and a member of the Presbyterian Church. My father was a Manipuri from a family of Krishna devotees and Sanskrit scholars. I grew up in a little hamlet in Shillong, where the population represented a fascinating religious and cultural melting pot. I had a ringside view of the various spiritual practices of the unconverted Pnar and Khasi people, the festivals, and the blood sacrifices performed to either ward off plagues and epidemics or cure someone of an ailment.

We also observed all our festivals—from Diwali and Holi to Easter, Id, and Christmas—with respect and enthusiasm. To top it all, I went to a Catholic School run by Irish nuns and fell in love with the rituals of the Catholic Church.

To my parents' alarm, I declared at age ten that I wanted to become a Catholic. Well, my mother told me I could follow any religion I wanted as long as I waited until I was sixteen. Eventually, following my cousin's advice, I was baptized in my mother's Presbyterian Church, but I was not happy, so I began calling myself a "protesting protestant."

Atheism and Modern-Day Prophets

Then, I fell in love with an atheist whose understanding of Jesus' teachings was so profound that I had difficulty believing his claims of atheism. I studied at the Yoga Institute, Santa Cruz East, in Mumbai. The course included the study of religious leaders, prophets, and mystics. The life of Jesus was a part of this study, and thus began my journey back to Jesus and my Church.

Then, I came across Sadhguru and Joyce Meyer. I love Sadhguru's view of life, humanity, the purpose of Yoga, deep belly laugh, and sense of humor. I love Joyce Meyer for making a significant difference in my way of thinking, my understanding of the Bible, and practicing being a Christian.

Spiritual Flexibility is an integral part of Patanjali's Yoga Sutras. This flexibility—practiced through the centuries—gives Indian culture the ability to assimilate different religious thoughts and beliefs. Thus, for me, too, this flexibility is about staying grounded in my faith and accepting people around me to practice what they believe. In summary, my kindness, goodness, and humanity do matter.

In this context, Spiritual Flexibility means:

- Humility or the ability to overcome my pride, ego, and opinions
- Acceptance of different perspectives and different ways of doing things
- Surrender—or letting go—exhibits strength, not weakness
- Ability to learn: a child-like curiosity and eagerness to learn something new

I remember one classmate at my Yoga institute proclaiming how she couldn't change her food habits. Our teacher went out into the garden, brought back a dry stick, and asked my classmate to come to the front of the class. "Bend this stick," our teacher said to my classmate, handing the stick to her. My classmate bent the stick, and the stick broke immediately. The teacher said, "When we can no longer accept or learn new ideas, we are as dry as this stick."

It was such a novel way of explaining a dead mind: a mind that had stopped growing and learning and had lost its flexibility.

The Lotus Stalk

Growing beneath the water's surface, the lotus stalk is slim yet strong. It moves this way and that when winds and water currents disturb the lotus beds. It accommodates the fish that swim in and around. It raises the flower above the water with great humility and generosity for the entire world to admire. We compare genuine beauty in a person to the lotus stalk. It is a flexible, strong, dependable, generous, forgiving, humble, and empowering person.

The Eightfold Path Patanjali's Yoga Sutras elaborate upon the asanas, a relatively healthy exercise. Anybody at any age can do the asanas and find them quite soothing. Yoga, however, is not only about asanas. While asanas help us attain physical fitness, we also need the Yamas and Niyamas. To do this, Patanjali collected all the ancient practices of Yoga into one treatise, Patanjali's Yoga Sutras.

There are Eight stages in Raja Yoga, also called Ashtanga Yoga or the Eightfold Path. Here, we must mention that the distinction between Kriya Yoga and Raja Yoga is not subtle: the former is more dynamic, while the latter is more intellectual. Both use asanas (Yoga postures), kriyas, bandhas, mudras, and shatkriyas, but Raja Yoga advocates involving the mind in these physical body exercises. Thus, Raja Yoga achieves more than any other Yoga practice. The Eight Stages are:

I. Yamas

1. *Ahimsa*

    Ahimsa, or non-violence, is the foremost Yama. The simple meaning of Ahimsa is not to hurt anybody. As we reflect upon this word, the deeper meaning of Ahimsa gains more clarity. It means not to inflict physical or mental pain on anyone, inflict violence on oneself, and not to cause suffering through our thoughts, words, or deeds. It also means not harming animals, plants, and our environment. Not getting adequate rest, doing asanas until we tire, beating an animal into submission, etc., are also forms of violence.

If we have lived life vigorously, we have had our share of disappointments, frustrations, anger, humiliation, sorrow, bitterness, successes, and pleasures. Often, we cling to these emotional hurts for years, waiting for the person (or persons) who caused them to admit their wrongdoing. At other times, we are just hungry for revenge! Unfortunately, the people who hurt us don't even remember what they did or don't care. They have continued to enjoy their lives while we have wasted precious energy and time (sometimes years) waiting for them to apologize or for our revenge.

When we are angry, we lose our peace and can become a giant pain to the few people who love us, such as our spouses, children, and caring friends. Being angry with ourselves is also violence we inflict upon ourselves! To find peace and joy, we have to be ready to change.

Change is hard! It is painful and requires sacrifice. In this context, 'pain' is of two types: the pain of change and the pain of staying in the same miserable state.

When I went to The Yoga Institute, I was dying for change, hungry, and ready to follow whatever they asked me to do. They surprised me when—on the first day—a teacher talked about the different aspects of Patanjali's Eightfold Path and introduced the concepts of Yamas and Niyamas.

For me, Ahimsa was a word I learned in History when King Asoka turned to Buddhism after defeating the King of Kalinga. Gandhi used Ahimsa to fight for India's Independence: how Martin Luther King Jr. led the Black people in their fight for equal rights in the United States of America and how Nelson Mandela won against apartheid in South Africa.

If the concept of non-violence could change the world, how could it not change my life?! I had to apply it to myself: I had to be kind to myself, love myself, and accept all the things I hated about myself. (I hated my upper lip, which has an operation scar. I was born with a harelip, and the corrective surgery went wrong when a nurse dressing the wound pulled a stitch and ruined the surgeon's effort to give me nice lips.) I hated my body because I was so skinny that clothes hung on me shapelessly. I couldn't think good thoughts about myself and take care of myself.

As I practiced Ahimsa, I felt better, and now I radiate positive energy to the world around me. Forgiveness is at the heart of most world religions and is quite evident in Ahimsa. It is difficult to say "Sorry," even when it is our fault. It is more challenging when it is not our fault, but we should take the first step. Taking that first step is extremely painful because I did it. My entire being screamed, "Why should I say sorry when they are the ones who have hurt me!"

The answer was powerfully insightful. I am doing it to free myself and get on with my life. When I "let go," "surrender," and "release" the pain, I live an infinitely happier life.

Forgiveness is not a saintly deed but a Yogic act for purely selfish benefit!

2. *Satya*

Satya or truth means not to indulge in lies and falsehoods. Satya means "reality." Telling lies compromises our integrity and complicates our lives; it changes reality and introduces a delusion. People who lie believe their lies with disastrous consequences.

Our lies also make us cowardly and weak; they weaken our souls and deprive us of our self-respect. It may seem we can achieve success only by lying, cheating, and corrupt means.

However, Satya will eventually catch up with such falsehoods and cause considerable discomfort. It is better to keep things simple by being truthful.

3. *Asteya*

This means non-stealing: To take something that is not rightfully ours, claim credit for work that we have not contributed to, or steal someone's idea and present it as our own—all these are stealing. Whether we are stealing a thing or an idea, it leads to a dilution of character. Simply put, to take anything without the owner's permission is stealing.

Asteya is honest in the material world. Rightfully establishing ownership over something (or stating our non-ownership over something) means Asteya. Since everything begins with me, I must introspect and admit that some things (or maybe many) that have gone wrong in my life are not someone else's fault. I have to take ownership of my faults. Even if things do not work out how I wanted, the past is over, and I must enjoy the present without worrying about the future.

4. *Brahmacharya (Abstinence from Sex)*

Some people take this to extremes, and you can see this even in religions where people of the Holy Orders abstain from sex all their lives. This is NOT Brahmacharya! This Yama informs you that if you overdo it, you may get bored! That's all! So don't believe the rubbish that says you must divert your sexual energy into something higher. Let us not forget that tantric sex or Vama Marga advocates many forms of sexual practices to achieve liberation.

5. *Aparigraha*

    Freedom from greed also means "Not to accumulate." Accumulation of things and cluttering the house with unnecessary stuff causes an imbalance in the physical environment and mental state. One is constantly worrying about one's possessions. The amassing of wealth can lead to illness of individuals, a sick economy, and a ruined environment. Unnecessary accumulation applies also to those who are unhealthy and diseased because of an unhealthy lifestyle.

II. Niyamas

Personal routines help save time daily. The following are self-explanatory:

1. *Shaucha* (Cleanliness)

2. *Santosha* (Satisfaction)

3. *Tapas* (Austerity)—Don't overdo it!

4. *Swadhyaya* (Introspection)—Have an awareness of your mind!

5. *Ishwara Pranidhana* (Surrender)—Many misinterpretations regarding this Niyama exist. This does not refer to surrendering

to God but to a higher form of yourself. Consider what Christopher Wallis states in *Tantra Illuminated*:

TATTVA #4: THE LORD (Īśvara) This is the level of the personal God, God as a being with specific qualities, that is, the Deity that can be named in various languages (whether the name is Krishna, Allah, Avalokitesvara, YHWH, etc.) This is the level of reality that most monotheistic religions presume to be the highest. Isvara is a generic, nonsectarian term for God. In Saiva Tantra, it is not only God who exists at this level; so do any beings who have reached that same awareness. Thus, the difference between Isvara and other beings abiding at tattva #4 is one of office, not nature.

When God becomes a synonym for every higher ideal, it removes the true meaning of phrases like Ishwara Pranidhana. Thus, this Niyama means to surrender to one's own higher consciousness. Please note that Isvara/Ishwara (God) is still three levels below what we can be!

III. Asanas

Yogic postures and exercises help create flexibility in our body and "tune" it for meditation. One should never practice pranayama without first doing the asanas and never meditating.

IV. Pranayama

We often understand this as breath control or breathing exercises. However, one should not think of the breath as air but as energy or life force. Prana means life, so controlling the prana is the basic idea behind any pranayama. It also helps the Yogi to concentrate during the initial stages of meditation.

V. Pratyahara

This refers to a "withdrawal of senses" wherein we are not always—compulsively or typically—engaged in our five senses. It is almost as if we are saying to ourselves, "There is more to life than what we experience through our senses." Practicing this kind of withdrawal is easy through meditation and facilitates advanced forms of meditation. It enables comprehension of our true nature by enhancing introspection.

VI. Dharana

Asanas and pranayamas prime our bodies so that concentration (dharana) can come quickly. There will be no physical disturbance as you maintain your posture and keep still. There will be no distractions from thoughts and memories. Additionally, you will focus on a singular idea or image for as long as possible. It is not unusual to get into a trance in such situations.

Sometimes, we achieve Dharana spontaneously when watching an exciting movie or reading an interesting book. This is meditation in action!

VII. Dhyana

Dhyana is the natural consequence of Dharana. This is when your contemplative state turns into a meditative state. From a neurobiological standpoint, one can say that more and more neurons are firing on a single idea or the object of concentration. One is no longer distracted—not even by one's wandering thoughts!

VIII. Samadhi

Stated Samadhi is achieving a union with the object of meditation. If the object of meditation becomes the infinite universe, then samadhi will achieve communion with it. It is evident that once you reach communion, there is no separation between the meditator and the object.

While you live, samadhi is seeing no separation from the external world. The highest level of moral achievement is seeing oneness with your enemy and, therefore, forgiving him. When you die, you become one with the universe's energy, going from one form of energy (as a human) to another (as cosmic dust)!

All this sounds quite grand! Moreover, I don't want to waste my time debating theories. If you prefer that you will ascend into heaven (or descend into hell), then that is your delusion of choice. You can assemble every Sunday, Saturday, Friday, or Tuesday with others who share the same delusion, and you will be blissful.

However, for many people, heaven-hell-god has become passé, and they seek a grander delusion that has the charm of being ancient and esoteric. It's in this context that Yoga comes to the rescue. Patanjali's Yoga Sutras and the Eightfold Path talk about samadhi as the ultimate achievement, but there are several stages before the ultimate stage.

A. Sabija Samadhi: This is meditation with a "seed object" as the focus of one's concentration.

B. Nirbija Samadhi: This does not use any object or a "seed idea." Concentration happens in the flow of thoughts, emotions, and feelings. This form does not distinguish between the things of the "flow" but focuses on the nature of the flow itself. In this state, one would say, "Why am I thinking these thoughts?" and NOT, "What are these thoughts I am thinking?"

C. Dharma Maha Samadhi: This state of consciousness does not see any separation between the thinker and the thought. One way to achieve this is to die: as soon as the brain is dead and the heart stops, the body unites with the material world, and there is no separation between the body, brain, and the inanimate universe.

We achieve it in another way when we experience dreamless sleep: we are in a state of samadhi. Now imagine you being able to achieve this state without sleeping or dying!

A. Sabija Samadhi

As we explore consciousness through these different meditations, we can see a further categorization:

1. *Samprajnata Samadhi (aka Savikalpa Samadhi):* Focusing on the different aspects of the seed object:

    a. *Savitarka Samadhi (Vitarka):* Focus on the object's physical attributes. Example: Different parts of a chair, color of the chair, etc.

    b. *Savicara Samadhi (Vicara):* Form, function, and essence of a chair. Example: Even without armrests, one can have a chair; a chair need not have four legs; the function of a chair can be a weapon when used to break it on a person's head!

    c. *Ananda*: Experience that different objects share one or more aspects: a cushion can comfort oneself or smother someone. The same physical features of an object serve completely different functions. We can sit on a pillow and a chair (completely different physical aspects serving the same function). Let's not forget that "happiness" is a loose translation of Ananda. It can mean the familiarity (and the comfort that the understanding brings) of knowing that entirely different things can serve the same function.

d. *Asmita*: This is the experience of a thing becoming something or turning something else. Example: A vague object becomes a rope on closer observation. When one gets more intimate, a string turns out to be a snake (or vice versa). A delicious-looking cake tastes like mud! Thus, expectations from an object come true (climax) or do not come true (anti-climax).

2. *Asamprajnata Samadhi (Nirvikalpa Samadhi):* When there is no object to concentrate upon, and instead, we have an idea to analyze, we experience a "sensation" between the different layers of analysis. It would be a mistake to think of this as going deeper or higher—it is more accurate to think of it as going into different dimensions! These are:

   a. Nirvitarka Samadhi: Vitarka to Vicara (Going from features of an object to facets of a concept)

   b. Nirvicara Samadhi: Vicara to Ananda (Going from facets of a concept to similarities between different images) Example: Communism and Capitalism both have money as the central idea. They may have opposite views on creating and distributing money, but they have money as the core philosophy. Contrast this to a society focusing on happiness as the core index of social existence (Bhutan).

c. Ananda to Asmita: All social systems have identical approaches to the same goal: happiness!

d. Transcending Asmita: One traverse from the "seed object" into Nirbija.

True Samadhi

No samadhi is possible without exposing oneself to the vagaries of life and everything it offers. In this sense, Tantra endorses the lifestyle of the Householder Yogi: one who takes part in all aspects of social and domestic life and continues his Yogic contemplation. They practice asanas by cleaning the garden and meditating by caring for a sick person.

As per Karma Yoga, they are a more remarkable Yogi than those who retreat to mountains and ashrams or forsake their social responsibilities to enjoy the isolation of ascetic meditation. They may claim to follow the Noble Eightfold Path, but nothing is noble about them!

Meditation can happen alongside the busy family life schedule; Kriya Yoga is possible within the plans of employment or running a business; mindfulness can be as simple as eating your meals without the distraction of conversation or checking messages on your Smartphone!

Layers of Ignorance

The path to samadhi unveils the layers of ignorance. When this happens, not only does one come highly near to God but also becomes God. On the way to samadhi, you will awaken your intuitive wisdom. This spiritual perspective is the nectar of immortality. In the deep recesses of the inner personality of a human being lie unlimited capacities, albeit as a seed. Instead of a "seed," imagine this as a coiled serpent, and you have Kundalini Tantra and the Chakra System that offer techniques to achieve samadhi.

Samadhi is the ultimate realization of the ego: from the supremeness of the "I" to the "I- ness" of the Supreme. There is no guy (or gal) in the sky! The subtle world is plentiful and boundless, and there are no constraints on our intelligence to fill this void. The tiny nature of meditative thought is as deep as the infinite facet of deep space.

There are no limits to blissful feelings at both ends of the spectrum. Similarly, deep meditation attempts to encircle both these boundless entities within consciousness. Here, the ego plays an important role: Someone with a healthy ego will contemplate the possibility of being as infinite as the universe and say, "I make this space meaningful by acknowledging its existence."

However, the ego-less person—in his timid humility—will say, "How can I be as big as the universe! I'm just a speck of dust!"

Religions preach the subjugation of the human mind to an external, omnipotent God. Thus, no religious person can ever attain samadhi!

Samadhi is within ourselves: it can take us from ordinary awareness to genuine consciousness!

Epilogue—Tantric Sex & Kundalini

No book on Tantra can be complete without discussing the Vama Marga as a pathway for enlightenment. This pathway (the Left-Hand Path of Tantra) uses esoteric sexual practices and rituals. The book also cannot be complete without discussing Kundalini Shakti and Kundalini Chakras.

The Vama Marga (Tantric Sex)

Tantric sex does not concern itself merely with sexual postures to please a sexual partner; it tells you how to please a lover. It ought to be clear that the distinction is not subtle! Love is Divine, but Lust is Pure! Sexual intercourse is only one form of communion between man and woman—a union of spontaneous energy that gives rise to the orgasmic response. In a sexual partnership, there is a state of bliss, an expression of love, passion, and joy.

The roots and traditions of the Vama Marga (Left-Hand Path) embraced sexual union and the satisfaction of the sexual urge as a form of attaining spiritual awakening.

What is Tantric Worship?

It is not only about sex, and it is not a religion. It is an intimate form of spiritual worship revering the feminine energy of the cosmos. This is like Eco-Feminism! In this worship, we don't connect with the divine/god; we merely connect with our own deeper self and sometimes even try to communicate with other beings.

If you are not in touch with your true nature, you will never be in touch with your true life purpose: a purpose you create for yourself. There is no exception to this rule. Remember, Tantra means "technique," which applies to all religions. There have been instances of Christian priests exploring these techniques to augment their spirituality. A former Jesuit, John Dupuche, who published *Towards a Christian Tantra*, exemplifies this.

Kundalini Shakti

Shakti (in Sanskrit) refers to the feminine energy of life that is constantly available to empower us. In Yoga traditions, there are three energies: the masculine energy (Prana), the life energy (Aditi), and the feminine energy (Shakti). This is similar to the Yin and Yang of ancient Chinese philosophy.

A Gift to Tantra

Tantra is a gift to Yoga, and Kundalini is a gift to Tantra! Kundalini is the "cradle of consciousness" corresponding to the pituitary gland—the grand controller of most other hormone-secreting glands. Kundalini Yoga is not abstract and mystical—it has definite physiological processes associated with it. The physical body is the foundation of everything sensational and spiritual.

Kundalini energy transcends the body, but it needs the body to manifest itself. Therefore, many Yogis have described Tantra as "that which deals with the body" or "of body." Remember, Tantra is not the spirit but a set of techniques that give us access to the spirit.

The journey of Kundalini's awakening happens through the Chakras. The literal meaning of the word chakra is "wheel or circle," but in the Yogic context, it is a spiral—ascending and descending simultaneously. Kundalini's awakening is not necessarily a spiritual awakening. People of different religions—along with their beliefs in God or gods—can experience a spiritual awakening in their own way. However, the Kundalini Awakening is available to all who undergo the path, even atheists!

Chakras and Nadis

Every human has many chakras, but Tantra only uses a few important ones. These chakras cover the entire "rainbow" of human existence, from the physical to the spiritual. The chakras are not in—or on—the spinal cord; they do not correspond to any vertebra! The location is purely symbolic but not abstract. These centers of awareness also control the functions carried out by the organs of that part of the body.

Similarly, the nadis are not necessarily the nerves. Sometimes, the nadis may correspond to the nerves, but their energy is subtler than that. For example, the interstitium is a network of fluid-filled spaces supported by a mesh of connective tissue. The medical community accepts it as an organ, the largest organ in your body. When required, the nadis use this as a passage; at other times, your breath would serve as a passage.

The Serpent

Kundalini is a primal power. In terms of modern psychology, it is the power of the subconscious mind. All higher-order creatures have a subconscious state, as REM sleep (Rapid Eye Movement) shows. You will also see your pet dogs and cats twitch in their dreams. Kundalini corresponds with the principle of Kali (the creative force).

In Shaivism, Kundalini is the Shiva lingam, the oval-shaped rock or pillar with a serpent coiled around it. We illustrate Kundalini as a resting serpent curled 3-and-a-half times. In all the oldest mystic cults of the globe, you will find the snake represented in monoliths and artifacts. This shows societies worldwide understood Kundalini (though they used different words).

Snakes fascinate humans because of the fear and the sense of grace they arouse. This fear/fascination is an instinctive trait found in all mammals! Additionally, it is a powerful symbol in all cultures of the world. A typical description of Kundalini stirring up:

"The snake awakens; it uncoils in Mooladhara and shoots up via Sushumna (the psychic passage), opening up the other Chakras as it travels upwards."

Having classified the spirit world into a hierarchy of spirits, Man knew that he could transcend his level and enter the domain of the angels and gods. Humans discovered the powerful prana (and prana Shakti) concept in this. In Tantra, he called it Kundalini.

Kundalini: Kali, and Durga

When Kundalini awakens but we cannot control it, we call it Kali. However, we call it Durga when we can handle it and use it for beneficial purposes. Kali is a female deity and the principal power of Kundalini. Some tantric traditions even consider her the ultimate achievement of the Kundalini Awakening (not Shiva). As the creative force, she catalyzes all creation in the universe.

Tantriks worship the cosmic power in its female avatar (because she stands for motion), and the masculine is the vast space. Remember that we are always moving: rotating, revolving, and falling. (Our entire galaxy is falling in the area!) Then, there is the emergence of Durga, the higher power, a more sophisticated and benign symbol of the subconscious.

Finally, I hope Tantra 2.0 has given you a glimpse into the beautiful aspects of your subconscious mind!

Book Preview

Coming soon,

Vigyan Bhairava Tantra: Conversations between Kali and Shiva

By Chaitanya Prabhu Hakkaladaddi

1. Kali speaks:

O Eternal One, I have attentively listened to the profound teachings that have emerged from the mystical union of Shiva and his Shakti.

I have also comprehended the sacred works, all the branches of Shakti, which encapsulate the essence of all knowledge.

2. Despite my deep understanding, my doubts persist even today.

What is your true nature, O Shiva?

Are you the decibel encapsulated within sound,

from which all magical mantras originate?

3. Can your true nature be realized?

Can a higher consciousness be achieved?

Is your infinite nature experienceable within a finite context?

Or does it suffice to comprehend all forms of Shakti (energy)?

These are my inquiries, O Shiva.

4. Is truth a manifestation of sound?

   If so, then which sacred syllable is it?

   Or can it be attained by focusing on the ascending psychic centers?

   I know the unstruck sound that arises without any vibration.

   Is that it?

   Or does it take the form of an eclipse?

5. Is your true nature beyond the infinite, even in intelligence?

   Or does it resonate with transfinite numbers?

   If it is experienceable, then you can't transcend the transcendence.

   And you are contradicted!

6. O Lord, if you are transfinite, beyond infinity,

   beyond form, pattern, color, sound, taste,

   then how is your experience separated from these?

   If you are the entirety of all that exists, you must contain the parts.

   Indeed, parts make the whole!

7. Through your wisdom, please dispel my doubts.

   Shiva responds,

   You are wise and complete in your knowledge.

   Your truth is perfect!

   Know now that you are delving into the occult nature of Tantra.

8. Dear One,

   Although this is the most secretive aspect of the Tantras,

   I shall reveal to you the teachings concerning the defined forms of Bhairava.

9. It all starts with the destruction of rituals.

   Every aspect of ritualizing me is empty of any spiritual value,

   like the entertainment we receive in nonsensical dreams,

   or the delusions of intense prayer and fasting.

10. Such are the practices of deluded intellects,

    who are trapped by scattered thoughts

    or inclined towards the performance of actions

    and meaningless, expensive rituals in their pursuit of meditation.

11. In truth, the essence of Bhairava is not found in any form,

    nor the flower offerings,

    nor the sacrificial animals,

    nor the three pathways of Kundalini,

    nor even within the manifestations of Shakti.

12. My proper form cannot be perceived,

    Period!

13. These descriptions of Bhairava's 'form'

    resemble scary stories told to disobedient children,

    or to trap those with immature intellect, to tread the spiritual path,

    just as parents entice their children with sweets.

14. Ultimately, no one can measure the state of Bhairava

    in terms of time, space, or direction,

    nor can it be defined by any attribute or label.

15. One can experience this inner state

    when the mind is free from modifications or thoughts.

    The true self of Bhairava, known as Bhairavi,

    is then realized as the bliss of one's inner awareness,

    a state characterized by completeness, devoid of contradictions,

    which encompasses the entire universe.

16. The essence of Bhairava's nature is pure, untainted,

    and permeates the entire universe.

Considering the supreme reality,

who is the object of worship, and who is to be appeased?

17. Thus, the transcendental state of Bhairava,

described and extolled,

is known through the absolute or highest form,

not as a Supreme God but as the Supreme Goddess.

18. Just as Shakti, the divine power,

is inseparable from shaktimaan, the possessor of power,

similarly, parashakti, the supreme authority,

who embodies the absolute and is identical with dharma,

can never be separated from Bhairava, the upholder of dharma.

19. Just as the power to burn is not separate from fire,

parashakti is not distinct from Bhairava.

However, in the initial stages, it is perceived as separate,

as a preliminary step towards attaining knowledge of its true nature.

20. The individual who enters into the state of Shakti

experiences a sense of unity with Shiva, without any division.

In this state, one truly becomes like the embodiment of Shiva.

In this context, it is said that Shakti manifests Shiva's essence.

21. Similar to how the flame of a candle

    or the rays of the sun reveal the existence of space, direction, and form,

    Shiva is shown through the medium of Shakti.

22. Sri Devi expresses: O, Lord of the Gods,

    who adorns Himself with a trident and skulls,

    please enlighten me about that state which transcends time, space, and direction,

    and is devoid of any distinguishing features.

23. Through what means can one achieve

    the state of complete fulfillment as Bhairava,

    and how does Paradevi, the highest form of Shakti,

    become the gateway to Bhairava?

    Please reveal this to me, O Bhairava,

    in a way that I can fully comprehend.

24. Shiva reveals: Paradevi, whose essence is creation,

    manifests as the upward prana (vital breath)

    and the downward apana (eliminative breath).

    By focusing the mind on the two points of prana and apana generation,

    the state of complete fulfillment is attained.

25. When the ingoing and outgoing pranic energies are restrained within their respective spaces without returning,

    the essence of Bhairava, which is inseparable from Bhairavi, becomes evident.

26. When Shakti, in the form of vayu (air) or pranic energy, becomes still

    and ceases to move swiftly in any particular direction,

    the structure of Bhairava emerges

    through the state of nirvikalpa (transcendental consciousness).

27. When kumbhaka (retention of breath) occurs

    after pooraka (inhalation) or rechaka (exhalation),

    the Shakti known as Shanta (peace) is experienced,

    and through that peace, the consciousness of Bhairava is revealed.

28. Concentrate on the Shakti that arises from the root chakra, mooladhara,

    like the gradually diminishing rays of the sun,

    until she dissolves in the twelve-petaled lotus at the crown,

    and Bhairava manifests.

29. Meditate on that Shakti as she ascends like lightning through each chakra,

    one by one until they reach the crown.

Then, at last, the glorious form of Bhairava dawns.

30. The twelve energy centers should be sequentially penetrated

    through a deep understanding of their associated twelve letters.

    By liberating oneself from the gross and the subtle realms,

    step by step, the Kundalini eventually merges with Shiva.

31. Then, after filling the tip of the crown

    and crossing the bridge between the eyebrows,

    the mind transcends all dualistic thought patterns,

    and the state of omnipresence prevails.

32. Just as one meditates on the five different colored circles

    on a peacock's feathers, focus on the five voids.

    Follow them until you reach the ultimate void,

    which becomes the gateway to enter the heart.

33. In this way, wherever there is mindful awareness,

    whether on the void or any other object,

    such as a wall or an esteemed guru,

    the blessing of absorption into the true self is gradually bestowed.

34. By closing the eyes and directing attention to the crown of the head,

    gradually stabilize the mind,

    and guide it towards the discernible goal.

35. Meditate on the inner space of the sushumna,

    the central axis of the body, the spinal column,

    which is as delicate as a lotus stem fiber.

    Through the grace of Devi, the divine form is revealed.

36. By utilizing the hands as instruments to block the entrances in all directions,

    pierce through the center between the eyebrows,

    and witness the bindu (subtle point of light).

    Gradually merging into it, the supreme state is realized.

37. Whenever one meditates upon the subtle fire,

    a state of agitation and trembling arises,

    followed by absorption and dissolution within the heart's cave.

38. The one who possesses the skill

    to listen to the unstruck sound in anahata (heart chakra),

    which flows incessantly like a rushing river,

    attains the supreme state of Brahma.

39. O Bhairavi, the one who repeatedly chants the Aum

    with unwavering focus on the void for extended periods

    experiences the vacuum itself,

    and through that void, the transcendental Shakti is revealed.

40. Whosoever engages in deep contemplation,

    even on the sacred syllables or letters of Aum,

    from the beginning to the end, in the form of emptiness,

    truly becomes one with the void.

41. As one's focused awareness is gradually established

    on the eternal inner sounds produced by various musical instruments,

    such as strings, wind, and percussion,

    ultimately, the physical body transforms into the supreme expanse of space.

42. By repetitively chanting and meditating

    upon all the gross sounds of the seed mantras,

    including the sound of 'M,'

    while immersing oneself in the emptiness within each sound,

    one truly merges with the divine essence of Shiva.

43. Simultaneously, all directions should be contemplated

    as expansive space or emptiness within one's body.

    The mind, devoid of all thoughts,

    dissolves into the vast nothingness of consciousness.

44. The one who contemplates simultaneously,

    on the emptiness of the spinal column,

    and the vacuum of the root,

    ultimately transcends all thought constructs.

    And achieves a mind devoid of attachments,

    empowered by an energy independent of the physical body.

45. Through steady contemplation on the emptiness of the sushumna,

    the void of the root, and the opening of the heart,

    one attains the state of nirvikalpa,

    wherein all thought constructs cease to exist.

46. Even a momentary concentration on the body as emptiness,

    with a mind free from thoughts,

    leads one to a state of thoughtlessness and, ultimately,

    one becomes united with the formless void known as Bhairava.

47. Focus your attention on all the constituents of the body,

    permeated by the expansiveness of space,

    so that the mind may find stability.

48. Contemplate the body's skin as a mere barrier

    or partition with no substance.

    Meditating in this manner makes one similar to the immeasurable void,

    which cannot be grasped through mundane meditation.

49. O embodiment of good fortune,

    through closed eyes and unwavering concentration,

    meditate upon the sacred mantra in the center of the lotus,

    within the heart's space,

    and thus attain the highest realization of spiritual truth.

50. When the mind dissolves into the space,

    between the eyebrows through unwavering awareness,

    and dedicated practice,

    the true essence of the ultimate goal

    manifests throughout the entire body.

51. By repeatedly bringing the mind to the space between the eyebrows,

    with utmost effort and whenever possible,

    the fluctuations of the mind diminish day by day,

    transforming each moment into an extraordinary state of being.

52. One should contemplate that

    the divine fire of time has consumed one's physical form,

    arising from the momentary existence.

    Eventually, tranquility will be experienced.

53. Similarly, by meditating with unwavering and focused attention

    on the entire universe being engulfed by the divine fire of time,

    that individual transcends ordinary humanity

    and attains a supreme state of being.

54. Concentrating on the constituents that comprise one's body

    and the entire universe,

    such as the fundamental elements and subtle vibrations,

    from the finest to the quietest,

    ultimately reaches the source of existence.

    This process reveals the supreme Goddess Paradevi

    at the culmination of meditation.

55. By meditating upon the gross and subtle energies within the twelve senses,

    one gradually refines them,

    ultimately entering the space within the heart and contemplating there,

    attaining liberation and freedom from worldly bondage.

56. Through contemplation of the entirety of the universe,

    and its evolution through time and space,

    the gross aspects dissolve into the subtle,

    and the subtle merges into a state beyond all forms,

    until the mind completely dissolves into pure consciousness.

57. By employing this method,

    one should meditate on all aspects and dimensions of the universe,

    leading up to the quintessential essence of Shiva.

    In this way, the experience of the ultimate reality arises.

58. O great Goddess, concentrate on perceiving this entire universe

    as nothing but boundless emptiness.

    By dissolving the mind in this manner,

    one attains the state of total dissolution known as laya (dissolution).

59. Fix your gaze upon the space within a pot,

    disregarding its outer structure.

    As a result, the pot disappears, and eventually,

    the mind merges entirely into the vast expanse of space.

    Through this dissolution,

    the mind becomes absorbed entirely in the emptiness.

60. Direct your vision towards a barren expanse devoid of trees,

    like desolate mountains or rugged rocks,

    where the mind finds no support to cling to.

    Then, the fluctuations of the mind diminish,

    and the experience of dissolution emerges.

61. Contemplate two objects in your thoughts,

    and when the knowledge of these objects reaches maturity,

    discard both and focus on the gap or space between them.

    By meditating on this void, the essence of experience arises.

62. With a restrained mind,

    concentrate solely on one object of awareness,

    letting go of all others,

    and preventing the reason from shifting from one to another.

Within this focused perception, awareness blossoms.

63. Concentrate with an unwavering mind on the entirety of existence,

    encompassing the body and even the universe,

    perceiving them all as nothing but consciousness.

    Then, the supreme consciousness emerges.

64. Through the fusion of both prana and apana vayus,

    whether within or outside the body,

    the yogi attains equilibrium,

    and becomes suitable for the proper manifestation of consciousness.

65. Simultaneously contemplate the entire universe,

    or your own body filled with the bliss of the self.

    Through this nectar of contemplation,

    one becomes alive with supreme delight.

66. Indeed, by engaging in religious austerities,

    great bliss arises instantly, illuminating the essence.

    But not becoming one with it.

67. By blocking all channels of perception,

    the pranashakti gradually ascends through the spinal column.

At that moment, sensing the sensation of an ant crawling within the body,

one experiences supreme bliss.

68. Immerse the blissful mind into the fiery manipura chakra

    in the middle of the fibrous lotus stalk of the Sushumna

    or the air-filled anahata chakra.

    Then, one merges with the remembrance of bliss.

69. Through union with Shakti, excitement arises,

    and ultimately, one is absorbed into Shakti. That blissful union,

    which is said to be the nature of Brahman, the ever-expanding consciousness,

    is, in reality, one's true self.

70. O, Queen of Gods,

    the bliss of a woman is attained even in the absence of Shakti.

    Bliss swells by fully immersing the mind

    in the experience of kissing, embracing, and cuddling.

71. When great joy is derived from any event,

    such as meeting loved ones,

    meditate on that joy with unwavering focus,

    until the mind becomes absorbed,

    and everlasting bliss arises.

72. By concentrating on the act of eating and drinking,

    and the pleasure derived from the taste,

    the contemplation of such enjoyment leads to a state of fullness,

    which then becomes supreme joy and bliss.

73. Through concentration on sensory pleasures,

    such as music or song,

    the yogis experience equal happiness and contentment within.

    By being fully absorbed, the yogi transcends the mind

    and becomes one with the supreme.

74. Whenever the mind finds contentment,

    and remains fixed solely on that contentment,

    the nature of supreme bliss reveals itself.

75. By entering the state preceding sleep,

    where awareness of the external world fades away,

    the mind becomes absorbed in the threshold state,

    illuminated by the supreme Goddess.

76. By gazing upon the space that appears,

    adorned with the rays of the sun or an oil lamp,

the true nature of one's essential self is illuminated.

77. During moments of intuitive perception, the attitudes of

    karankini, krodhana, bhairavi, lelihanaya, and khechari are unveiled.

    Thus manifesting the ultimate attainment.

78. Seated on a soft cushion, using only one buttock,

    with the hands and legs in a relaxed position,

    at this moment, the mind becomes filled with transcendence.

79. Direct your gaze within this space by

    assuming a proper posture and curving the arms and hands into a circle.

    Through this practice of absorption,

    the mind attains peacefulness.

80. The seeker must maintain an unwavering gaze,

    devoid of blinking upon any object's external form.

    When the mind becomes fixated and detached

    from all other thoughts and emotions,

    it immediately attains the state of transcendence,

    the divine consciousness of Shiva.

81. By placing the middle of the tongue on the wide opening

    and directing consciousness to the center,

    mentally repeating the sound "Ha,"

    the mind dissolves into a state of tranquility.

82. Whether sitting or lying down,

    one should envision their body as weightless

    and suspended in the vast expanse of space.

    Through this practice,

    the mental constructs and patterns of the mind gradually diminish,

    freeing it from the burdens of past experiences.

83. O Divine Goddess,

    through the gentle swaying or rocking of the body,

    one attains a serene state of mind

    and merges into the flowing stream of divine consciousness.

84. O Devi,

    by fixing the gaze unwaveringly upon the clear sky without blinking

    and maintaining a steady awareness,

    one immediately achieves the nature of Bhairava, the supreme reality.

85. The seeker should contemplate the sky

    as the embodiment of Bhairava

    until it becomes fully absorbed within the forehead.

    Then, the essence of light permeates that entire space,

    existing in the state of Bhairava.

86. Having gained an understanding of duality,

    the interplay of light and darkness in the manifest world,

    one who can once again experience the boundless form of Bhairava

    attains enlightenment.

87. In a similar vein,

    one should contemplate the terrifying darkness of the night

    during the dark fortnight of the moon

    if one aspires to attain the form of Bhairava.

88. Likewise, with closed eyes,

    one should meditate upon the profound darkness that spreads before them,

    recognizing it as the form of Bhairava.

    Through this practice, they merge with that darkness.

89. Whoever can restrain even a single sense organ

    attains the singular void devoid of duality.

    In this state, the self is illuminated.

90. O Devi, through reciting the sacred syllable "A,"

    in the absence of the dot and the final sound,

    a vast flood of knowledge regarding the Supreme Lord, Parameshvara,

    arises instantaneously.

91. When the mind merges with the final sound, the visarga,

    it becomes unsupported and transcendent.

    In this way, the reason is touched by the eternal Brahma,

    the supreme consciousness.

92. When one meditates upon one's self,

    visualizing it as a boundless space expanding in all directions,

    the mind becomes suspended, and the divine energy, Shakti,

    in the state of consciousness,

    is revealed as the proper form of the self.

93. Initially, one should lightly pierce a limb of the body

    with a sharp needle or any other instrument.

    Then, by directing consciousness towards that point,

there arises a movement towards the pure essence of Bhairava.

94. Through such contemplation,

    the inner instrument of the mind, the Antahkarana,

    and other constructs cease to exist within oneself.

    As a result, one becomes liberated

    from the limitations imposed by mental constructs.

95. Maya, the illusory principle

    residing within the manifested existence,

    gives rise to names and limited activities.

    By contemplating the nature and functions of the various elements,

    one realizes their inseparability from the supreme reality.

96. By observing the desires that arise fleetingly,

    one must end them.

    Through this practice,

    the mind becomes absorbed in the source of those desires.

97. The seeker should contemplate,

    What remains of myself when my desires fail to produce proper knowledge?

    By immersing oneself in the essence of one's being

and identifying with it,

they become one with that essence.

98. Whenever desire or knowledge arises,

    the mind should steadfastly focus on it,

    recognizing it as the essence of the self.

    By making the mind one-pointed in this manner,

    the seeker realizes the fundamental nature of the elements.

99. Compared to absolute knowledge,

    all relative knowledge lacks a cause

    and thus, becomes baseless and deceptive.

    In reality, learning does not belong to any individual.

    One becomes united with Shiva, the ultimate truth,

    by contemplating this.

100. Bhairava, the embodiment of undifferentiated consciousness,

    resides within all forms.

    Those who contemplate the entirety of creation

    infused with this consciousness

    transcend the limitations of relative existence.

101. When the inner manifestations

of lust, anger, greed, delusion, arrogance, and jealousy are observed,

fixating the mind upon them,

the underlying essence alone remains.

102. One attains happiness

by meditating upon the world of appearances,

recognizing its illusory nature

akin to a magical spectacle or a painting,

and perceiving the transience of all existence.

103. O Divine Goddess,

the mind should not dwell upon the sensations of pain or pleasure.

Instead, one should seek to understand the essence

that resides between these opposing forces.

104. By relinquishing attachment to one's physical form,

one should contemplate with a resolute mind,

realizing the omnipresence of the self.

The perception of separateness dissolves through concentrated insight,

leading to profound joy.

105. By contemplating a specific knowledge,

   such as the analogy of a jar,

   or recognizing that desires and their ilk exist not only within oneself

   but permeate the entire cosmos,

   one becomes all-encompassing.

106. The interplay between subject and object is familiar to all.

   However, yogis remain vigilant in their awareness of this relationship.

107. Contemplate one's consciousness,

   both within one's own body and within the bodies of others.

   Gradually abandoning all expectations tied to the physical realm

   expands one's awareness to encompass all.

108. Liberate the mind from all attachments

   and abstain from indulging in the fluctuations of thoughts.

   In doing so, the self merges with the supreme self,

   attaining the state of Bhairava.

109. The Supreme Lord, omnipresent, omniscient, and omnipotent,

   is none other than oneself.

I possess the exact divine nature as Shiva.

Firmly contemplating this truth,

one becomes united with Shiva.

110. Just as waves arise from the ocean,

    flames from a fire,

    and rays of light from the sun,

    the waves of Bhairava give rise to the diverse emanations of the universe.

    Undoubtedly, these waves originate from within oneself.

111. By spinning the body in circles until it collapses upon the ground,

    the energy that was once in a state of agitation becomes tranquil.

    Through this cessation, the supreme condition manifests.

112. When unable to perceive objects

    due to ignorance or distorted perception,

    if one can dissolve the mind

    by absorbing it into the erroneous perceptions themselves,

    then, after this absorption-induced stillness,

    the form of Bhairava emerges.

113. Listen, O Devi, as I reveal the secrets of this mystical tradition.

By fixing the eyes in an unwavering gaze without blinking,

the state of kaivalya, absolute liberation, arises instantly.

114. By closing the openings of the ears and the lower orifices

and meditating upon the inner palace of the unstruck sound,

one enters the eternal realm of Brahma.

115. Standing atop a deep well or abyss

and gazing steadily into its depths,

the mind becomes devoid of all fluctuations,

and dissolution promptly manifests.

116. Wherever the mind may wander,

whether outward or inward,

the all-pervasive state of Shiva follows.

117. Wherever consciousness directs its attention

through the channel of the eyes,

by contemplating upon that object alone,

recognizing its inherent similarity to the supreme reality,

the mind merges and experiences the state of wholeness.

118. At the beginning and end of a sneeze,

> in moments of terror, sorrow, or confusion,
>
> when fleeing from a battlefield,
>
> during intense curiosity,
>
> or upon the onset or satiation of hunger,
>
> the external manifestation of Brahma is revealed.

119. When the mind is set aside,

> and memories of significant past experiences,
>
> such as one's homeland or birthplace arise,
>
> rendering the body supportless,
>
> the omnipresent and mighty Lord manifests.

120. O Divine Goddess, in a fleeting moment,

> when one directs their gaze upon an object and slowly withdraws it,
>
> an awareness and understanding of that object arises.
>
> In this process, one becomes a vessel for emptiness,
>
> a dwelling place for the void.

121. The intuitive knowledge

> that emerges from the profound devotion of an entirely detached person

is known as the Shakti of Shankara.

By regularly contemplating upon this Shakti,

the supreme consciousness of Shiva is revealed within.

122. When one perceives a specific object,

all other things fade into emptiness.

The mind finds tranquility and rests peacefully by contemplating this emptiness,

even though the particular object is still known or perceived.

123. What may appear as purity to those with limited understanding

holds no concept of purity or impurity for those who have experienced

the divine essence of Shiva.

The natural purification, known as Nirvikalpa,

transcends all conceptualizations

and leads one to attain true happiness.

124. The ultimate reality of Bhairava exists everywhere,

even within ordinary individuals.

By contemplating, "There is nothing other than Him,"

one attains a state of non-duality,

where awareness becomes homogeneous.

125. The one who does not discriminate between friend and foe,

honor and dishonor,

recognizing Brahman as complete and all-pervading,

attains supreme happiness.

126. One should never perceive others as friends or enemies.

Free from such distinctions,

the nature of supreme consciousness,

the essence of Brahman, blossoms within.

127. One ultimately realizes

by contemplating Bhairava as beyond comprehension, knowledge, grasp,

and imagination.

128. By fixing the mind upon the eternal, unsupported, vast,

omnipresent expanse of outer space,

one enters into the formless and unmanifest dimension,

which defies estimation or calculation.

129. Wherever the mind may dwell,

casting it aside at that moment,

it becomes unsupported and free from disturbances.

130. The term Bhairava signifies the dispeller of fear and terror,

   the one who roars and cries,

   the one who bestows all,

   and the one who pervades the entire manifest and unmanifest universe.

   By continuously repeating the word Bhairava,

   one merges with Shiva.

131. When asserting, "I am,"

   "This is mine," and similar notions,

   the mind becomes unsupported through inspired meditation on Tat,

   the highest reality.

132. By contemplating every moment on the eternal words,

   omnipresent, unsupported, all-pervasive, and master of the universe,

   one attains fulfillment through their profound meaning.

133. This world is illusory, like a magical illusion,

   devoid of any true essence.

   What essence can be found in magic?

   Firmly convinced of this,

   one attains inner peace.

134. How can there be knowledge

   or activity of the changeless self, the atman?

   All external objects are subject to the control of knowledge.

   Thus, this world is empty and void.

135. There is neither bondage nor liberation for me.

   These concepts only frighten the timid

   and are mere reflections and projections of the intellect,

   just as the sun's image is reflected in water.

136. All sensory experiences bring forth pain and pleasure

   through contact with the senses.

   One abides in one's true self by relinquishing attachment to sensory objects

   and turning inward, withdrawing the senses.

137. Knowledge unveils all, and the knower is the self of all.

   One should contemplate that

   the ability and the knower are inseparable and one.

138. O Beloved One,

   when the mind, awareness, energy, and individual self,

   these four components dissolve into nothingness,

   the state of Bhairava manifests.

139. O Divine Goddess,

   I have briefly shared more than one hundred and twelve ways

   through which the mind can be stilled,

   devoid of any surge of thoughts.

   By knowing and practicing these methods, people attain wisdom.

140. The state of Bhairava is attained

   when one is firmly established in any of the one hundred and twelve dharanas,

   and through their words, they possess the power to bestow blessings or curses.

141. O Divine Goddess,

   even by practicing a single dharana,

   the seeker becomes liberated from the confines of old age,

   attains immortality,

   and is bestowed with extraordinary powers.

   They become the beloved of all yoginis and the master of all Siddhas.

142. The Goddess inquired,

   O great Lord, if this is the nature of the ultimate reality,

   the seeker is liberated while still alive

and remains unaffected by worldly affairs when engaged in action.

143. Thus, the Devi asked, O great Lord,

please explain to me in the proper sequence which should be invoked

and how the invocation should be performed.

Whom should one worship or meditate upon,

and how can one please the deity through such worship?

144. Continuing, Devi inquired,

To whom should the invocations be made?

And to whom should the offerings be presented during the sacrificial rituals,

and how should these actions be performed?

Sri Bhairava replied These acts are merely external forms of worship.

145. Engage in contemplating the supreme consciousness repeatedly;

this itself is a form of japa.

The spontaneous sound produced within oneself

is undoubtedly the essence of the mantra.

Such japa is to be practiced in this manner.

146. When the intellect becomes steady,

    formless and devoid of any support,

    then true meditation is attained.

    Imagination of the divine form with physical attributes

    such as body, eyes, mouth, and hands,

    is not true meditation.

147. Offering flowers and other objects

    is not the true essence of worship.

    Instead, stabilize the mind in the vast expanse of the great void,

    transcending thoughts in a state of nirvikalpa.

    It is from this reverence state that the mind's dissolution occurs.

148. By being firmly established in any of the practices described here,

    the experiences that arise from such practices gradually develop daily

    until absolute fulfillment is attained.

149. Proper oblation is offered when the elements, senses, and mind

    are poured into the fire of the great void,

    Bhairava, or the supreme consciousness,

    using consciousness as a spoon.

150. O Supreme Goddess Parvati,

    in this sacrificial offering characterized by bliss and fulfillment,

    one becomes the savior of all beings by eradicating sins.

151. The most profound contemplation

    is to merge oneself into the Shakti of Rudra.

    Otherwise, how can one worship that element,

    and who is it that is to be pleased?

152. One's self is undoubtedly the all-pervading bliss of liberation

    and the essence of consciousness.

    Merging into one's nature or form is considered the natural purification bath.

153. The worshiper who worships the transcendental reality is the same.

    Therefore, what is this worship?

154. Prana and Apana, moving swiftly in specific directions

    by the desire of Kundalini, the great Goddess,

    extend themselves and become the supreme pilgrimage site

    for both the manifest and the unmanifest.

    155 One who diligently pursues and abides in this sacrificial offering, filled with supreme bliss,

attains the ultimate state of Bhairava

through the grace of the divine Goddess.

The breath is exhaled with the sound 'Ha,'

and inhaled with the 'Sa.

Thus, the individual continuously repeats

this particular mantra, Hamsa.

156. As previously mentioned, this repetition of the Divine Goddess's mantra

should be practiced twenty-one thousand six hundred times daily and night.

It may seem accessible to some but challenging for the ignorant.

157. O Goddess, this most profound teaching,

which leads to the state of immortality,

should not be disclosed to anyone.

158. These teachings should not be shared with other disciples,

with those who are wicked,

or with those who have not surrendered to the feet of the guru.

They should only be revealed to advanced souls

with self-control and minds free from distractions.

159 and 160. Those devoted disciples of the guru,

who, without any doubt or hesitation,

have renounced their attachments

to family, spouse, relatives, home, village, kingdom, and country

should be accepted for initiation.

The worldly possessions are all temporary, O Goddess,

but this supreme wealth is eternal.

161. One may even sacrifice one's life force,

but this teaching, the nectar of the highest order,

should never be abandoned.

The auspicious Goddess said,

O Great Lord Shankara, God of Gods, I am delighted.

162. Today, I have comprehended absoluteness, its essence, and the heart's innermost core of all the Shaktis.

163. Thus, the Goddess, being steeped in delight, embraced Shiva.